ANIMAL Chakra Healing

Bringing Balance, Health, and Joy to Our Animal Companions

Joan Ranquet

FINDHORN PRESS

Findhorn Press
One Park Street
Rochester, Vermont 05767
www.findhornpress.com

Findhorn Press is a division of Inner Traditions International

---

Disclaimer
The information in this book is given in good faith and is neither intended to diagnose any physical or mental condition nor to serve as a substitute for informed medical advice or care. Please contact your health professional for medical advice and treatment. Neither author nor publisher can be held liable by any person for any loss or damage whatsoever which may arise from the use of this book or any of the information therein.

Cataloging-in-Publication data for this title is available from the Library of Congress

ISBN 979-8-88850-261-7 (print)
ISBN 979-8-88850-262-4 (ebook)

Printed and bound in the United States by Lake Book Manufacturing, LLC

10 9 8 7 6 5 4 3 2 1

Edited by Susan Kemp
Cover photo: ID 156181857 © Famveldman | Dreamstime.com
Illustrations by Becky MacPherson
Text design and layout by Yasko Takahashi
This book was typeset in Adobe Garamond Pro, Nicholas, Agenda, Malila, and Supria Sans

To send correspondence to the author of this book, mail a first-class letter to the author c/o Inner Traditions, One Park Street, Rochester, VT 05767, USA and we will forward the communication, or contact the author directly at **https://joanranquet.com**.

Animal Chakra Healing

"Joan Ranquet is a master animal communicator, energy healer, and teacher. Her book *Animal Chakra Healing* should be on every animal lover's and veterinarian's shelf. It is easy to read, fun as well as scientific, and very informative. As a holistic veterinarian, I use the energy of the chakras every day. The more we understand about chakras and healing, the healthier all animals will be. 11 Stars and 5 Paws up!!"

—**JILL TODD, DVM, CVA, CVCP**, holistic veterinarian

"A superb deep dive! *Animal Chakra Healing* offers not only a comprehensive primer on the chakras but goes beyond in teaching how to assess and then balance chakras for our beloved animal friends. Joan Ranquet's series of practical questions, chakra by chakra, encourage the reader to explore both the behavior and dynamics of their pet as well as their own unspoken feelings, shedding light on behavior issues and illuminating solutions. This book serves as a guide to truly see things from an animal's perspective, which Ranquet feels is the key to making a real difference in their lives, their health, and their happiness . . . and ultimately in ours. A fascinating must-read for both animal lovers and those interested in spiritual development, personal empowerment, and the practical application of the rich system of chakras."

—**MARGARET LYNCH RANIERE**, coach, trainer, and author of *Unblocked* and *Tapping into Wealth*

"Animals carry emotional energy, just like we do. They feel grief, fear, and even joy in ways we often underestimate. In *Animal Chakra Healing* readers are given a kind and thoughtful guide to understanding the deeper energetic life of animals—especially how imbalances in their chakra systems can impact their health and behavior. This book beautifully affirms what I have seen time and time again: that healing is possible when we address the root energy imbalances. If you have ever sensed that your animal companion was holding on to something unseen, this book will guide you in helping them feel safe, balanced, and loved."

—**Dr. BRADLEY NELSON, DC Ret.**, energy healing expert and author of *The Emotion Code*, *The Body Code*, and *The Heart Code*

"Just as humans have chakras, so do our animals, and learning how to keep them cleared and balanced can work wonders on behavior as well as emotional and physical health. *Animal Chakra Healing* provides all a person could even need to understand and balance the animal chakra system. It's a must-read for any animal lover looking to understand and assist their pet in living the best life possible."

—**TAMMY MASTROBERTE**, spiritual teacher and author of *The Universe Is Talking to You*

"*In Animal Chakra Healing* Joan Ranquet beautifully blends her decades of experience as an animal communicator with the wisdom of chakra energy. With clarity, compassion, and practical tools, she helps readers—whether they're new to chakras or seasoned in energy work—connect with their animal companions on a deeper level. A heartfelt and insightful guide for anyone seeking greater balance, health, and joy for the animals they love."

—**TAMI TOMLINSON**, creator of Canine Chakra Yoga

"Joan Ranquet opened the door to animal communication, and people are amazed at the power this unleashed. After we learn we can communicate, then we need to know how to interpret the messages we receive. This book is a vital stepping stone in that ascendant communion. Lots of answers await inside. Pick it up. Crack it open. Follow the path, and may you never be the same!"

—**Dr. RICHARD E. PALMQUIST, DVM, GDVCHM, ACCHVM**, integrative veterinarian and past president of the American Holistic Veterinary Medical Association

"*Animal Chakra Healing* has helped me enormously to understand what each chakra really is, what it does, how it affects humans and animals, and how it plays out in the world at large. It has helped me to truly understand my own rescued animals at The Gentle Barn, how their past traumas manifest in their bodies, and how to heal the related chakras. Joan, thank you for writing this book and for your brilliance!"

—**ELLIE LAKS**, founder of The Gentle Barn and author of *My Gentle Barn* and *Cow Hug Therapy*

"Now and again, I have been asked—and have asked myself—the obvious question: Why animals? There's no simple answer. I'm curious about animals. They amuse me. They keep me company. They're nice to look at. I think I have the same response to animals that I would if Martians landed on Earth. I would like to get to know them and befriend them, all the while knowing we were not quite of the same ilk. They seem to have something in common with us, and yet they're alien, unknowable, familiar but mysterious."

—SUSAN ORLEAN, *On Animals*

CONTENTS

PART ONE: THE EIGHT CHAKRAS

PART TWO: SOLUTIONS

PREFACE

I was fascinated with chakras since the first time I heard about them in a yoga class at the age of 17. I couldn't really get a true grasp on this concept. As I deepened my meditation practice, there they were again, chakras. They were so exotic, yet to hear a westerner speak—the over-simplified meanings left me a little disappointed in the explanation I was given, leaving me hungry for more.

By the late 1980s I was living in Los Angeles, with my theatre degree, my acting training from NYC and the UK—I had stars in my eyes. I would eventually write screenplays, do a ton of theatre and some odd film work here and there . . . only to end up becoming an animal communicator.

Many people who end up working within the intuitive circles are first drawn to the arts because it is a community of outliers. Arts reflect the world, society as a whole and culture. Empaths can get pummeled by the world, until they find that north star.

My own personal gravitational pull was to the animals and that is where I landed and grounded eventually. It always was and continues to be the north star for me, my mission and purpose. Meanwhile, my journey to find my anchor, my pull, my own purpose was a circuitous, painful—yet fun—route full of laughter and my own healing.

While I should have been at weekend workshops on acting and such, rather, I was learning Tellington TTouch (a type of bodywork for animals) and attending workshops by such luminaries as Barbara

Ann Brennan and Rosalyn Bruyere. And more, I was doing sweat lodges, working on healing horses with geodes during a full moon by the Los Angeles River, while a sweat lodge was happening simultaneously offering healing prayers led by my friend, Butch Artichoker of the Lakota Sioux in South Dakota. I mean, I went all in with the healing thing.

And it kept coming back to learning more about chakras. The Bodhi Tree Bookstore was within walking distance of my apartment. It was a mecca for all things world religions, metaphysics, intuition, and more. I found myself there weekly. I devoured *Hands of Light* (Bantam, 1988) by Barbara Ann Brennan, and Rosalyn Bruyere's book *Wheels of Light* (Fireside/Simon & Schuster, 1989). I was hooked. In fact, from here I can see the *Hands of Light* book, it is so tattered, it is almost broken in half. It became like a bible for me when it came to horses with injuries, diseases, and more.

As I transitioned over to becoming an animal communicator and leaving my film world union dues behind, energy healing took on an even bigger role in my life.

I have always been one to meditate, workout, and ride or hike before anything happens in the day. In the 80s and 90s that meant driving to the barn where I boarded my horse(s). On the drive, I listened to audio tapes—yes, I said it, tapes—and one that I drilled into my head all the way from West Hollywood to Atwater Village in Los Angeles was Caroline Myss' *Anatomy of the Spirit: Seven Stages of Power and Healing* (Bantam, 1997). I can still hear her Chicago accent as I come up over Los Felĺz with the Sierras lightly covered in snow in the distance. The brilliance of what I was hearing was accented by the early light and the beauty around me. I would have an enlightened time with my horses and drive all the way back, now through massive traffic, and wouldn't even notice because her words had me transported.

As my own animal communication practice was taking off and my medical intuition was blossoming into being something unique—especially for horse and rider—I was thrilled to hear that Caroline Myss and Dr. Norman Shealy were putting together a medical intuition course in St. Louis.

And so, I signed up. And then I signed up for the Ph.D. program in Energy Medicine. I was in the program for a little over a year when in 2000 I had to drop out due to getting married, taking on step-kids, and the busyness of life. But I loved every second of being in that energy, the energy that I and select friends embodied on our own. To be in a ballroom with 250 other people was thrilling.

My big challenge in that program was that I had to translate everything from human to animal, without a veterinary degree. Things like Energetic Psychopharmacology was super great, and tryptophan was a great alternative to Prozac but was it going to show up in a blood test in the horse or dog show ring? That could ultimately get the animal disqualified as if they were drugged. Some herbs would be fatal for cats, some minerals were of no help to dogs. I had some hurdles in the program.

I kept separate notebooks for dogs and cats and another one for horses. My brain exploded because there weren't volumes of information for animals. Fortunately, Dr. Shealy and his wife had horses. Mary Charlotte Shealy was a Centered Riding instructor, so gaits, motion, health, and well-being were everything to them. And so, each day after class I practiced privately with Dr. Shealy and his horses, and he reviewed my notes and correlations.

While I never finished that degree, I never stopped taking notes, looking for patterns, formulating ideas, typing up stories, and filing it all away—in a very big notebook. It is fun to revisit all the research I did and mingle with the stories I wrote up years ago.

Some of this book is metaphorical, some of it is allegorical, and there are big overarching themes around each chakra and animal. What I always say to my students is thateven if we are looking at the pattern of the chakra regarding an animal, we are still looking at an individual. We always want to make room for the unique character standing before us.

I am dedicated and driven beyond measure to help humanity understand that animals have souls, they have big feelings, purpose, karma, wounding, healing, and their lives have meaning. Animals are part of our family. Nature and wildlife are cousins in a larger familial ecosystem. Animals are not commodities; they are living beings who deserve agency. It is the underlying theme to everything I do, whether it is a private one-on-one session with a client about their animal, teaching in my school Communication With All Life University (CWALU), any speaking event, including my TEDx talk, and each of my books that I've authored. It colors every minute of every day that I enjoy my animal family as they express their essence and beingness in their daily lives as part of a multi-species family.

This mission is layered into every word of this book. As long as one species (or many) are oppressed, our collective well-being is out of balance. The sooner we see animals as their own beings, the sooner we will elevate the whole world.

INTRODUCTION

WHAT IS ALL THIS CHAKRA TALK?

Wheel, lotus, vortex, all of these describe the word "chakra." In this mysterious history of the chakra's origin, what we have come to know through the Indian Vedic texts, Upanishads, or through the Tantric lens is that the physical body has energy centers. The number of centers is as mysterious as the origin of the chakra. The Buddhist texts mentioned four or five, whereas the Hindus believed six or seven. The number of chakras goes up to 114. Twelve chakras is bandied about by some schools of chakra-thought but most agree upon the traditional seven chakras in the body.

This chakra system was also found in ancient Greek, Egyptian, and Chinese cultures. Traditional Chinese Medicine has invisible maps known as the meridians that run throughout the body system, connected to the organs and emotions. It is believed that the Native Americans had a system; the Pueblo Nation was said to have a connection to the Creator and the Earth and several vortexes in between.

Worldwide, ancient cultures recognized mental, physical, emotional, and spiritual aspects to our lives and that intuition and creativity was involved also. They recognized that there needs to be balance and flow. This was largely done through yoga, mantras, prayer, breathwork, meditation, and visualization.

If you are completely new to energy and chakras, imagine the physical body with spinning wheels or discs, like a vortex, a whirling, three-dimensional mass, or a cone-shaped funnel extending from the body. Chakras are located in the physical body, along the spine that extends outward beyond the body. The chakras are associated with areas and organs in the physical body and with themes. Think of it this way: each chakra, in either you or your animal, holds specific information based on individual history, and it also contains the potential of what each chakra represents.

Chakras categorize our experiences for us throughout the body. If we are facing a challenge, dynamic or shift in our mental, physical, emotional, spiritual, sexual, and financial world, it could be because of something inhibiting the corresponding chakra from being in its full power to groove and flow. There are behavioral, relationship, and health consequences if we are not maintaining a balance. I like to think of chakras as different, interrelated theme parks that are owned by the same company. Or even better, like distinct, beautiful national parks in one state.

Traditional chakras have symbols associated with, and representing, each one. See the human chakra system with symbols below (and on the color plate).

1. Muladhara: "Root" – base of the spine
2. Svadhishthana: "Where the self is established" – sacral/under the belly button

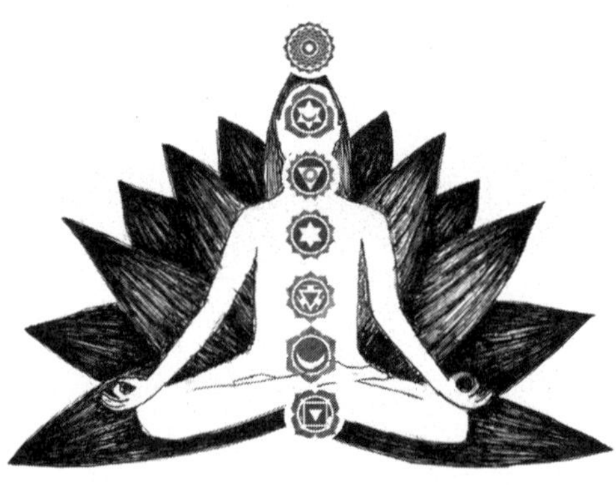

Fig. 1: The human chakra system

3. Manipura: "Jewel City" – solar plexus
4. Anahat: "Unstruck" – heart center
5. Vishuddha: "Purest" – throat center
6. Ajna: "Command" – brow/third eye
7. Sahasrara: "Thousand-Petaled" – crown

For humans, conscious thought, clearing techniques, intention, and a healthy lifestyle can keep the system balanced. For animals, this is up to us as their stewards. Without balance, there seems to be a disruption in their behavior, relationships, or health. As an animal's emotional leader and human companion, it is our duty to keep an eye on, or feel into, what might need a little chakra shake-up to restore balance and harmony.

Evolution of Our Understanding

One thing became clear: the physical aspects of the chakras were actually connected and coordinated with the nerve centers and the endocrine system. H. P. Blavatsky and other theosophists became intrigued and introduced the chakras to the Western world. Associations were made with the physical body as Charles Leadbeater recognized the chakras as a true system. Carl Jung integrated this system into his work. Psychic Edgar Cayce integrated the chakras into his dream state work. In the 1990s, Dr. Norman Shealy, Caroline Myss, Rosalyn Bruyere, Barbara Ann Brennan, Dr. Valerie Hunt, and more were bringing the work to the forefront.

In 1994, Dr. Valerie Hunt released a series of music and sound tapes called The Music of Light, in which the frequency of each chakra is harmonically coordinated to the field of energy known as the aura. Now chakra music and attunement through sound and vibration is very common. Mantras introduced us to that notion. Chanting *Om* (Aum) can raise the frequency of the third eye and crown chakra, and the symbol of *Om* can balance all the chakras.

In many ways, the frequency of the chakra knows no words. When balanced, it reverberates in a fine-tuned world like the perfect note from a violin. Imagine the cello representing the root chakra and moving up to the crown to hear a harp with a chorus of angels singing. Literally sounds, thoughts of the sounds, and even the energy alone can realign the whole system in a matter of moments. Like anything else, when out of whack it is discordant.

I feel very fortunate that in the early 90s, I found myself at weekend workshops with Rosalyn Bruyere, Barbara Brennan, and any acupressure, TTouch or any hands-on course for horses I could find. I came across Gary Douglas and Access Consciousness before it became what it is today. In the early 1990s, healing was a hobby until about the mid-90s and then this "hobby" coincided with my busy life as an animal communicator and became part of the menu of services I offered.

My friend Susan Davis started teaching something called Bioscalar Wave Therapy created by Dr. Valerie Hunt. It is a technique that I simply call the scalar wave, which involves running the energy, clearing the chakras and bringing in a scalar wave to rearrange the cells into a coherent field of energy. Susan was very close with Dr. Valerie Hunt and became her number one teacher of the technique, as well as her resource for data on the chakras, the energy field, and physical "dis-eases."

I became riveted with this technique and became Susan's right-hand person every Saturday morning as every week she taught this course to people who were struggling with their health, emotional crises, and more. During the week I then experimented with the technique on my animal clients. I went on to become Dr. Valerie Hunt's main resource for the data on animal chakras, the animal's energy field, and animal "dis-eases."

The success I had with animals balancing the chakras and bringing in the scalar wave was off the charts. I watched tumors shrink, bacteria dry up, bloodwork change, energy restored to elderly dogs, cats, and horses—and even behavioral issues transform, and so much more.

In 1998, I became approved by Dr. Valerie Hunt to also teach the Scalar Wave and have been teaching it ever since. Chakras are a very important aspect to this healing process, so when I teach this class, I always spend time giving students a baseline of the chakras.

I continued to take notes and file the amazing stories. I searched for information on animal chakras in the 1990s and the only thing I could find was Diane Stein's *Natural Healing for Dogs and Cats* (Crossing Press, 1993). That book sits on my shelf along with Barbara Ann Brennan's *Hands of Light* (A Bantam Book, 1988) and Rosalyn Bruyere's *Wheels of Light* (Atria Books, 1994). Each book is a treasured vessel of love and is as tattered, loved, and in as many pieces as Ted Andrews' *Animal Speak: The Spiritual & Magical Powers of Creatures Great & Small* (Llewellyn Publications, 1993). These were my true resources.

I went on to study with Dr. Norman Shealy and Caroline Myss for a Ph.D. in Energy Medicine, with a focus on medical intuition. When Dr. Norman Shealy tested my DHEA, he said I had the highest DHEA in any human my age he had ever seen. I knew it was from the scalar wave and chakra work. I never finished the Ph.D., but I continued to strengthen my file of notes based on working with those great teachers. I did continue to send information to Dr. Valerie Hunt. She was set to create the first aura-meter but sadly died before the machine was finished.

The aura, and the connective "tissue" between herds, prides, packs, and flocks was ever present in my mind. I could go to a barn full of horses and as I facilitated the scalar wave on one horse, all the horses were nodding off—not in a full hypnotic sense—with releases coming out of every orifice. This was as real as the computer I'm typing on now.

As much as I loved just sticking to the seven traditional chakras in my classes, I started understanding more about the eighth chakra, the "Soul Star" that we are all connected to and is also known as our connection point to the God/Divine/Universe/Spirit/Source.

Dr. Rupert Sheldrake released his book *Dogs That Know When Their Owners Are Coming Home* (Crown, 1999) and introduced, in scientific terms, the idea that many ancient cultures subscribe to the morphic resonance. The term morphic resonance denotes a field of energy created that living organisms can tune into and develop according to the intelligence, emotions, and identity of that field. Of course, that field is connected to a much bigger field—THE FIELD—if you will, meaning the all-encompassing big field of God/Divine/Universe/Spirit/Source. And quantum fields. Meanwhile, every home, flock, herd, tribe, family, pride, culture, and pack has its own signature ecosystem that has a morphic resonance in which individuals can be autonomous yet also part of this field of energy.

I started working with the idea that the eighth chakra for animals was their ecosystem, their morphic resonance, their own field of energy connected to the bigger field, and of course the biggest field of God/Divine/Universe/Spirit/Source. In many ways, the eighth chakra represents the home of instinct that we humans have dulled. Everything that comes into the body comes into the field first and informs either our thoughts, emotions, or chemistry how to respond or react. To me it made sense to call it the eighth chakra.

Meanwhile, on the other side of the pond, in England, international animal communicator and healer Margrit Coates was also researching on the animal chakra system and discovered the animals' eighth chakra, for which she is credited worldwide. She shares her amazing findings in her books *Healing for Horses: The Essential Guide to Using Hands-On Healing Energy with Horses,* and *Hands-on Healing for Pets: The Animal Lover's Essential Guide to Using Healing Energy,* published in 2001 and 2003 by Rider/Penguin Random House.

Chakras have been evolving forever and will continue to do so. It seems that everyone has their take on it. Whether it is physical, emotional, spiritual, archetypal—energetically, it is all fascinating. Once we learn it, we start to see it in everyday life, such as the salt-of-the earth, first-chakra man with a deep voice that fixes your car tire and disappears as quickly as he appeared. Ovulation becomes a very second chakra phenomenon, as does giving birth to a human, a book, a business, and so on. When we don't listen to our gut, our third chakra, we get sick to our stomachs. We can literally have heart pain when we have a broken heart. We lose our voice when we can't seem to express ourselves—a very fifth chakra experience. We might associate migraines with what we aren't seeing with our third eye. And we've all seen that seventh-chakra person who seems to walk on air as they bat their ephemeral eyelashes. We've all met that person who wears their heart on their eighth-chakra sleeve for the world to help.

Creating a personal system for yourself becomes vital in the pursuit of learning about the chakras. Once you start seeing chakras, you can never not see them. In yoga it is common to have heart-opening poses like Camel Pose (healing the heart chakra), or Tree Pose to ground the Root Chakra. Mantras, exercise, prayer, joy, gratitude, energy healing, bodywork, and singing (even if off key) can realign the chakras.

Creating an animal chakra log through the notes you keep on and for your animals becomes helpful in developing a better understanding of them. Understanding animal chakras brightens our ability to see animals as beings with souls, karma, wounding, healing, and a trajectory and purpose that may or may not have anything to do with us. By taking this bird's-eye view, each chakra gives us a crystalline glimpse into what makes up each individual being and how we might restore balance with and for them.

How to Read This Book

The beginning eight chapters reflect the first eight chakras and include location of the chakra, color, and what organs/emotions are associated with it. Descriptions have been broken into:

- Symbolism
- Species-specific/breed-specific
- Shadow side
- Chakra organs, systems, structure, and meridians
- Emotions and energetics
- Behaviors, dynamics, and relationships
- Stories

As you go through these chakra descriptions, highlight or take note if something resonates with you about your animal. In the following chapters, we will put it to work! Chapter 9 explains how you can tune in to the animal chakras and offers questions over questions. In Chapter 10 you find information on healing the chakras, including assessment charts and a balancing technique. Chapter 11 is full of outside ideas to support the health, happiness, and wellness of your animal companion(s).

Get your long fins and put your snorkel on, we're going deep!

Enjoy!

PART ONE

THE EIGHT CHAKRAS

THE CHAKRA SYSTEM

The full chakra systems of cats, dogs, horses, chicken, and humans are depicted on the color plates in this book.

THE FIRST CHAKRA—SURVIVAL

"In the ancient mysteries, each chakra was said to be the seat of the body. The first chakra or kundalini chakra is the seat of the physical body, the generator of the physical reality as each of us experiences it. In other words, the first chakra makes life. It makes all physical form: my physical form, your physical form, and others' physical forms as well. This chakra holds the very mystery of life (animated physical form) as well as the drive for procreation. Maintaining physical life is its most basic function."

—Rosalyn L. Bruyere, *Wheels of Light, Chakras, Auras, and the Healing Energy of the Body*

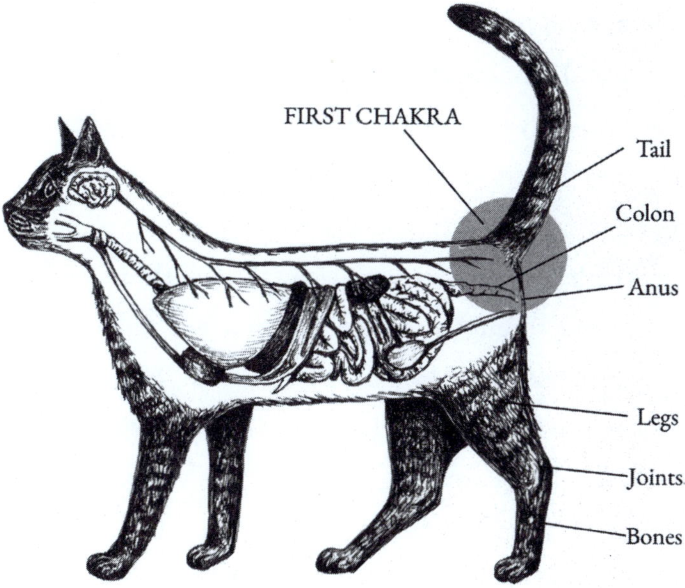

Fig. 2: The first chakra (root chakra)

The Great Migration—The Drive for Survival

One of the greatest moments or movements in the wild is the great migration. The wildebeests start this trek in search of greener pastures, literally. As the momentum builds, they leap off the sides of riverbeds *en masse* and trample through rivers, stepping on each other like concert goers. Wildebeests have another name, gnu. The name comes from this weird nasal moo sound that they make while their hooves beat the ground as their crusade ensues. Zebras are pulled in their wake. They say that zebras like to eat the top part of long grasses, and the wildebeest really mow down to the roots. Synergy indeed. They are perfect grazing partners.

The thundering sound, the collective drive, the change in the air also attracts predators. All the big cats await in the grasses for a baby, a weak one, a slow mover. Crocodiles camp in the river and have their pick as their perfect prey is on parade.

Nearly two million animals participate in this journey. Nearly 250,000 will die throughout this endeavor, either by predator, drowning, or other accidents. And many babies are born during this time, babies that are literally up and running in minutes.

In part, the weather sparks this run; in part, it is the desire for the perfect grasses. Yet there is something else that motivates this myopic drive: instinct.

Fossils have been found to suggest the wildebeest has been on this east African route through the plains for over one million years. Originally, this mission was fueled by a need for survival. While it may or not be the case now, it is built into the DNA, the muscle memory of the individual, the cellular memory of the species, and deeply encoded into the morphogenetic field of the ecosystem.

The Great Migration is a classic first chakra activity. A collective action passed down through ancestors, this herd, and the DNA of the species.

Cue Gloria Gaynor now for "I will Survive." Okay, there's no disco ball in the wild, but there is plenty of survival going on. We can have a little fun with chakras!

Anodea Judith suggests that there are elements to the chakras, and that the first chakra is the earth element. The great migration creates a great clockwise circle (chakra) from Tanzania back up and around to Kenya through the seasons. This need for survival literally creates and obeys a well-trodden deep path. This path serves as a chakra in the earth.

The Power of That Hind End, the Take-Off in Flight

The hind end makes up the first chakra. We will go into more first chakra anatomical details in a moment. Many animals, certainly the domestic animals, we will be discussing throughout this book are quadrupedal, meaning that they operate on four legs. Reptiles, birds, and some of our aquatic friends—including mammals—are tetrapods. Tetrapods have four limbs, or are descended from animals with four limbs, and they have evolved to perfect their locomotion and survival.

As the story of evolution goes, about 400 million years ago, a lung fish emerged with strong enough pectoral fins to support him/herself on land. For some, these fins eventually became limbs and we evolved into reptiles, birds, amphibians, and mammals.

A tetrapod and a quadrupedal have four limbs. A tetrapod is Greek for four "feet" (limbs) and quadrupedal is Latin for four limbs. It can be confusing. But quadrupedal denotes that all four limbs are used for locomotion.

A seal is a perfect example of a tetrapod. Somewhere through development or not developing, it lost the need for four feet and is able to move from land to sea and back to land again. A pigeon is a tetrapod. A whale is a tetrapod, we humans are a tetrapod (aka bipedal).

An alligator, a zebra, a dog, cat, horse, and even infant humans crawling are considered quadrupedal.

While sixty percent of the body weight is carried in front for a quadrupedal, their lift-off is in the hind end. Imagine this first chakra body part. The hind legs activate like first responders, all based on the instinct, drive, or thought of the being. Sometimes the hind end responds before thought.

The gaits of a quadrupedal are broken into walks, trots, canters, and gallops. The need to survive is a gallop, whether predator or prey.

The gallop is driven by the strike-off of a hind leg, propelling the front end into motion. As the hind leg lands and strikes off again, the body is in suspension. The hind end starts the motion, and it goes on its own volition once the rest of the body responds. This is what I will refer to as the engine of the body.

Imagine, herd activity is powered by the first chakra; fight or flight is fueled by the first chakra. Most play is fired up by a launch from the hind end.

This hind end action propels many activities:

- A cat will squat down and leap. The landing often involves the hind end tucking under and landing with equal grace to the front end.
- A dog jumping differs a bit in that the lift-off comes in the front end but the propulsion—again, think engine—comes from the hind end. They land on their front end.

- A bird's flight starts from a leap from their feet. In the case of waterfowl, they still use their strong legs and webbed feet to create the thrust forward for flight.
- Whales and dolphins use their tail for propulsion, and as a propeller to navigate.
- Apes and monkeys can go between bipedal and quadrupedal movement, using their knuckles as they amble along—but it starts from those hind legs.

First Chakra Symbolism

Chakras, particularly the first chakra, are associated with the Kundalini energy moving through the body, up through the chakras. This energy is referred to as a female serpent, coiled in the root chakra, ready to spring up the spine. Through each of the chakras this energy goes, bringing awakening to each area—chakra—and ultimately as it reaches the seventh chakra, consciousness and enlightenment arrives. This first chakra is the seat of that expanding life force.

Some would argue that animals are already conscious and enlightened. Science would say the opposite. Like all things, the truth is somewhere in the middle and rather than assigning the entire animal kingdom with "enlightenment" we look at individuals. Besides, whether animals in general have reached enlightenment is not the discussion at hand, but the life force springing forth certainly is.

For that reason, wildebeests springing off riverbanks into the unknown epitomizes the life force at work. The first chakra is all about physicality. And the earth. And grounding. The primal need for survival. Power in numbers—herds, prides, packs, pods, flocks, etc. The first chakra is also about loyalty, justice, and belief systems.

The great wildebeest migration is all of that:

- Survival—better grass
- Loyalty—loyalty to what we learned when we were just moments old
- Justice—we have a right to this land
- Belief systems—this is what we do!

Ultimately, this chakra symbolizes and embodies survival. When that is threatened, it results in fight, or flight.

In the world of human chakras, the first chakra represents tribe, family, family of origin, family bonds, family secrets, belief systems sent down through the ages (DNA), traditions, family habits, and family quirks. The first chakra governs the emotional/mental body, mental health, and logic. This is where our unfinished business sits.

In the animal kingdom, the first chakra represents the herd, flock, the pride, the pod, the colony, the murder, the coalition . . . the family of origin, the family characteristics, and the family quirks. The power in numbers is essential for the survival of a herd.

Instinct + Structure + Hierarchy = Safety

While animals survive and thrive on instinct, the ecosystem creates structure, seasons, the terrain to navigate, daytime, and nighttime.

For a predator:

- There is the "territory."
- This is the way we hunt.
- Always try to single out one from the herd.
- Don't get injured as this can be your demise—stay away from hind feet of prey.

For prey:

- This is how we camouflage.
- Here are the safer areas.
- Stay together.
- Look to the leader and/or your mom.
- Band together with others once you are a juvenile.

These given circumstances create structure and hierarchy within the herds, flocks, packs, prides, and pods. Instinct with structure creates safety. Animals who are solo and are establishing territory learned all of this from their mother in growing up. The hierarchy creates safety and a deeper understanding of self and the role that the individual plays in the greater good. Nothing could be truer for our animals at home as well.

Important messages also are delivered *in utero*. Animals who are feral but around humans often get the message before they are born not to trust humans. Feral cats, mustang horses, dogs on the street, and more.

Often that "coding" in the feral animal's software known as their psyche, heals through generations, just as humans do. We see generational healing and evolution as people overcome things that their parents were unable to. The same can be said for that little kitten that came out of a third-generation feral colony. She might be timid at first with humans, yet brazen. And may eventually become the lap cat. Maybe.

Feral is different from wild. Feral has been rewilded. At one point, they were domesticated, so deep back in their DNA is a more interactive experience with humans. In other words, they aren't as suspicious, tentative, and sometimes as aggressive as our wild cousins might be.

The first chakra is also associated with the environment. The environment, whether it is a territory for wildlife or a new home for a dog from the shelter, becomes a dynamic force in the development of the persona. It can be the opportunity for an animal to blossom, or a space that compounds old damage, trauma, and wounding. Through established relationships, clear boundaries, and a calm household, an animal can settle in and blossom easily.

Equally, an animal can associate a space that compounds existing damage. For example, imagine a cat came from a home where it was picked on by the other cats and now faces a pair of tough siblings. It might revert immediately to its shy self, finding all the same sorts of hiding places. Suddenly the cat is a victim of circumstance and the environment again and is unable to live in its full potential.

Adaptation becomes part of the unspoken dialect as wildlife moves from territory to territory during seasonal changes. When our domesticated friends get adopted, they too become masters of adaptation. Newly adopted animals often "audition" for the first six months in their new home. The real personality and quirks usually come out after a period of assessment, and they settle into their new life.

Unfinished business is a first chakra phenomenon. It can get transformed through lifetimes or ancestry. Where we see it playing out is in the end stages of life. We can see an older frail animal who is suffering from some sort of disease go into what I call a "state of grace" where they literally test out the waters of the other side while keeping a foothold in this world. People wonder what is keeping them here. Many people believe that they are "hanging on" for their human. I would venture to say that they are working through their unfinished business. Often this includes creating completion with the other animals in the household. Or perhaps an ongoing telepathic connection with their previous guardians. Of course, their current humans are part of this final phase.

First Chakra Species-Specific/Breed-Specific

For humans and animals alike, the first chakra is about all that we've inherited. For animals this is largely about genetics. What traits they've inherited. And how this plays out with their soul's contract, as well as the contracts with the others in their world—humans and other animals.

Like humans, animals come in with soul contracts. Those contracts include curriculum. The contracts and curriculum may or may not involve other souls. In other words, their soul has been informed through the species, through the breed and then through the persona on what needs to be carried out with a divine stamp of approval. The evolution of the lesson means complete integration of the soul, the persona, and the divine. If the "job" isn't fully realized, it can be carried over into the next lifetime, though it may or may not look similar at all.

For example, perhaps someone's soul needs to experience an extreme of being aloof with a desire to connect. What better form to play that out than showing up as a "look but don't touch" type of cat. Better yet, a Gemini cat!!

Imagine it was time to experience extreme loyalty, coming in as a dog that barks from a perch on the back of a couch at every person, animal, and leaf that passes by the window.

Imagine a soul who has the complexity of needing to experience a mix of wild and confined moments—showing up in this lifetime as a horse would do it.

Imagine needing to be gracious with confinement, coming back as a domesticated bird would be perfect.

And of course, imagine needing to come back as a being whose instinct has been overridden by logic. Well, that would be the human experience!

Nature-invented adaptation and animals have followed suit. Notice the heavily driven freeway overpasses with all the pollution dropping down directly on the fresh flowers that are budding.

Watch a palm tree dance in a hurricane, or look closely at the subtle life that springs forth after a riverbed has dried up. A fallen log or stump becomes a nurse log, providing a home for so much more life to flow out of it, such as mosses, lichens, small bushes, and trees! Survival all the way.

Loss of habitat due to climate change has resulted in grizzly, polar bear hybrids. As water was less available, camels went for longer periods of time without water. This behavior created a physiological shift so that the hump developed to store fat and reduce the need for water.

Domestication

Domestication hardly changed the cat much. All of our cats are descendants of either the mummified cats found in Egyptian tombs, African wildcats, and cats from Asia. As the rodents were drawn to the cradle of civilization—Mesopotamia—agriculture and civilization were developing, so were the cats. Humans and cats lived closely together as the cats kept the rodents away from the crops.

The Egyptian cats came on the scene a little later and had a more tame and friendly demeanor. Other than cat coats, there is not much difference in the DNA of your house cat to some wildcats.

All cats fall under the *Felidae* category. There are 41 species. There is a split between big and small cats.

Technically, cats domesticated themselves for survival. Like dogs, they are opportunists. Unlike dogs, it took roughly 9,000 years for them to jump in our laps. Okay, I may have exaggerated. But you get the gist if you have a cat. Even though they are more aloof than dogs, they are the most popular companion for homes.

One key differentiation is that as the domestication process began with dogs, they were selected to do certain tasks. These diversified characteristics and activities led to the various breeds we see today. And the cat would argue, they—cats—didn't need to be counted on for tasks as they were already "purrfect." As a result of this self-awareness on the part of the cat there are roughly forty-five to forty-eight cat breeds. Whereas there are over 400 dog breeds.

The domestication of wolves and jackals certainly changed as they became dogs. As some dogs came closer and closer to the cave, others stayed very clear of humans and maintained their suspicion, high alert, and even aggression. The suspicious dogs stayed in the fight or flight survival mode and stayed wild. The dogs that moved closer, got closer and closer. These "dogs" stayed next to the cave or settlement and eventually moved in. This created a little ease for the survival game for both man and dog. In some cases, early on, these "dogs" actually partnered up with humans for hunting.

They say dogs did their own genetic manipulation, but we went a little over the top, breeding them for specific characteristics. Of those 400 dog breeds, the dog's pleasing manner, opportunism, and willingness to adapt to new levels, plus man's evolving needs created modern dogs.

It isn't a completely sinister anthropocentric movement that we have engineered this many breeds to suit our every need. Both humans and the developing "dog" alike enjoyed the loyalty, companionship, and protection that this new "dog" provided. As the dog took ownership of their new role, these traits were enhanced. And humans, whether it was the birth of the agricultural era, industrial revolution, or the Victorian era, started manipulating the gene pool.

Then man started breeding for traits:

- Hunters needed a good sniffer for hunting.
- Hunters needed great sight to see prey.
- The nineteenth Century brought on designer dogs as Victorian women loved the companionship of smaller dogs.
- A dog with a big bark was a great protector.
- Webbed toes, a soft mouth and a charming personality created the perfect hunting companion as retrievers cheerfully retrieved waterfowl from chilly waters.
- Herding dogs exhibited patience and courage and were tasked with guarding the flock or the herd.
- Working dog definition is to "assist humans."
- Big-boned dogs could pull carts.

And ultimately, conditions were imposed upon them by humans and that is why we have four-hundred dog breeds. I bring that up because—for them to survive—we have to help them develop more, sustainably, if you will. With interbreeding, we could be breeding our domestic animals into extinction like our wild cousins.

The Shadow Side of the First Chakra

What inbreeding has done – just to name a few:

- The dalmatian—deafness and hip dysplasia
- The German shepherd—degenerative myelopathy, hip, and elbow dysplasia

- The cocker spaniel—hereditary eye problems, ear problems, and allergies

And our breeding for compliance has not been a favor to the beagle. Their characteristic kindness and expressive eyes mark them to be the chosen breed for testing in laboratories. This unbearable cruelty is a direct result of our tendency to breed for our best interests and not theirs.

As man continued to perfect breeds for their own needs, we have then gone on to vilify these very breeds that we have created.

Especially the following breeds:

- Doberman
- German shepherd
- Rottweiler
- Pit bull

All the things that we love and hate about dogs have been superimposed upon them by human needs. Again, as discussed earlier, there are some dogs and cats who seem to choose to be domesticated, and have evolved side by side with us. And some of those purse dogs certainly seem to be grateful for their free ride.

Canini that fall under *Caninae* comprises of:

- Gray wolf and many wolf species
- Coyote
- Domestic dog
- Jackals
- Dingo
- African wild dog
- Dhole (Asia)
- Fox

Both the domestic dog and domestic cat can be either predator or prey depending on their environment and/or their age. Both dogs and cats saw fit to domesticate themselves for survival.

The horse is a different story altogether. They always have been, and always will be, prey.

The domestication of horses was a lot more dramatic. Meaning, it wasn't their choice. The domestication of the horse is believed to have happened as early as 4,500 BCE. Archeologists have discovered this through their exploration of tomb burials filled with both horse bones and chariots.

Some of these early, domesticated horse species lived in the Eurasian Steppe area, which extends for 8,000 kilometers (close to 5,000 miles). The word steppe means unforested grassland. This area extends east to west from the mouth of the Danube River, almost reaching the Pacific Ocean. To the north, forests from European Russia, Siberia, and Asian Russia create a boundary. There is no clear boundary to the south but there it becomes very dry, fading into the desert.

The Eurasian Steppe was the precursor for the Silk Road, a lot of trade and back-and-forth activity between humans happened here. This area experienced nomads, hunter gatherers, and early agriculture. And this is where the domestication of farm animals, including the horse took place.

The Steppes was a natural fit for grazing animals, particularly horses who are "monogastric hindgut fermenters." They prefer grass but the northern borders of the steppes would provide some bark, leaves, and roots. Equines—horses, donkeys, and zebras—spend 60 to 80 percent of their time grazing, depending on the terrain.

There is always an argument about domestication. Did it start when they were tamed and interacting with humans? Or did it start when man controlled their breeding?

All equines are social and live in groups. Usually, the territory is spoken for by a stallion and the rest of the herd is harem style. It is made up of several mares, females, and their offspring. Equines tend to be nomadic. Because they are social, it is believed that they were slowly domesticated by taking the foal and raising it with humans while the mother was slaughtered. Foals did well with humans.

The Tarpans and the Przewalski's horse remained wild. The Tarpan is now extinct, and the Przewalski's horse has been brought back from near extinction, and lives in Mongolia. What we consider "wild horses" now—like the mustang in America, the Brumby of Australia, and the Dartmoor and New Forest of the UK—are feral. They have been rewilded. There are over fifteen feral horse colonies in the world.

Archeologists have found equine bones with chariot pieces and art. It is thought that horses were domesticated and used to drive the chariots and carts that crossed the Steppes in invasions from Europe to Asia, and vice versa. It was the nomads of the Steppes living on pastoral land—managing the grazers—that are said to have simply hopped on the horse and created quite a synergy between horse and rider. This changed everything for man, as it simplified warfare. It also changed everything for the horse.

As they were domesticated, like the dogs and cats, they were bred based on temperament. This created the perfect horse for warfare, sport, work, entertainment, and culture. Yet, to see horses— whether out in the wild or in a small paddock—grazing with their heads down, and the wind lightly blowing their tail in the breeze is true peace. As a result of their peace and an individual's steady temperament, horses are used for therapeutic purposes. They have been bred for temperament, speed, endurance, agility, strength, and more. Through time, this has changed physiology and created over two-hundred different breeds.

Horses were broken into three categories by temperament and build, not temperature:

- The Cold-blooded—which have developed into draft horses, the working horses—were known for their big bones, and capability due to size and their calm, patient nature.
- Hot-blooded horses were originally called "oriental horses" and were hotter natured. Meaning, they have a lot of get up and go. They are "light" and agile. Their bones are finer. They are "spirited." They came from the eastern part of the steppes. The gene pool of most of the lighter horses come from the Arabian horse. Hot-blooded would also be high fight or flight.
- The warm-blooded—which came more from the Europe Forest part of the Steppes—has developed into a breed or breeds. When crossed with thoroughbreds and Arabians, warm-blooded horses became carriage horses, and war horses. Though they are a combination of cold-blooded and hot-blooded horses—big bones and smaller bones—their refinement has made them best known now for riding and has developed into sports, such as dressage and show jumping.

The Bedouins were known to selectively breed and create the Arabian as we know it now. The desert was highly uninhabitable, and man and horse had to endure it. The Bedouin tribes kept their breeding private, and the lineage was kept as pure as it could be. Records were by memory and shared throughout time verbally.

The horse's symbolism is that of power, speed, and grace for many cultures. Once you took horses away from the grazing area, and kept them in unnatural settings, it became more costly to feed them. This resulted in horses being assigned the symbolism of prosperity and higher status. Prosperity and higher status are not just for the more civilized, this status was also seen in indigenous cultures across the lands. Horses became currency. The Bedouins considered the horse to be a gift from Allah that should be cherished.

The Ecosystem as a Metaphor

Right now, our ecosystem is under duress and in survival mode. We are experiencing the wrath of a planet in an imbalanced overdrive due to overpopulation, consumerism, and carelessness. In many ways, this fast-paced unraveling of the ecosystem is reflected in the struggle for survival of many of the earth's species. The imbalance has resulted in overpopulation in animal shelters, which is answered by the genocide of epic proportions of dogs and cats as well as others. In the US and Australia, the "wild" horses are being rounded up and killed to "protect the nation's public rangelands." Most of this is fueled by—in the US—the Cattlemen's Association; they would like open space for their cattle, who will eventually be consumed. That very same consumerism is a death sentence for wolves, coyotes, and cougars, a.k.a. human/wildlife conflict.

First Chakra Organs, Systems, Structure, and Meridians

The first chakra color is RED! The ROOT chakra. Survival. Rooting us all back to our beautiful Planet Earth! Whether a tetrapod, bipedal, or quadrupedal, these legs and/or tails are the life force in fight, flight, freeze, or flee.

Organs and Systems

The first chakra is the home of our sexual organs and of male hormones—"our" meaning all species, including humans. The first chakra rules reproduction, as the organs are here to procreate and, of course, it governs the bones, joints, and the anus. It's also worth repeating that the first chakra also includes the legs or hind legs, the feet, the tail, and the fluke!

- Physiological systems at work here: Immune—fights diseases
- Endocrine systems at work here: testes
- Nerve plexus: inferior hypogastric plexus—network of nerves of the pelvic cavity—and the coccygeal plexus
- Spine: coccyx, base of tail

The first chakra sits at the base of the spine. We humans are sitting on our first chakra. Our legs could act as deep roots, grounding us. For the quadrupedal (four-legged), it is the hind legs. For the bipeds (two-legged), such as humans, birds, kangaroos, some primates, and more, it is simply the butt and legs. For both bipeds and quadrupeds, the first chakra also includes (hind) legs, feet, hooves, paws, claws, and webbed feet. For tetrapods, the first chakra represents the tail, the fluke.

All tetrapods are limbed fish. Most are land-living vertebrates such as frogs, turtles, whales, and snakes. Through time, they have lost some of their limbs. Because of their ancestry, they are still considered tetrapods. Many original tetrapods are now considered quadrupedal.

This space at the base of the spine is also the base of the tail for animals. Tails are a splendid thing. We see a cat with a flat tail and a flat back, moving like a hovercraft across a room to hide and we know they are in fear. If a cat is angry, one or two flicks of that tail and we all know to get out of claw reach. Dogs tuck tail and drop their hind end. That hind is ready to run or launch to protect if need be. Horses say "talk to the tail" as they literally swing their hind ends around so fast, it could clock you and before you know it, you're having a dirt breakfast. Our cetacean cousins use that tail to power into hyper swim, while using it as a rudder to navigate the fight or flight.

Tails tell a tale. You could spend your life reading tails and it would be all you would need to know about what level of comfort an animal is experiencing. It is a true warning. Think of the rattle on a rattlesnake. An overstimulated reactive dog will often wag their tail as if they were eager to see you, and then that hind end springs to action. A horse being ridden will engage their tail in agitation if it is not going well, or it will sit calmly if they are calm.

Our finned friends (mammals, tetrapods) have an area called the peduncle, located between the first and second chakras that is the base of their spine as the body moves into the fluke. The definition of peduncle is "the main stalk." In botany, a peduncle supports a flower. With our cetaceans, it supports the distance between the organs, the spinal structure, and the actual fluke (end of the tail). This distance is a soft tissue miracle as it has no bones and is made up of muscles and fiber. It is so powerful that it can propel a dolphin up to 30 miles per hour or toss a humpback whale into the air. A dolphin can swim on its side, on its stomach, in deep waters, upside down, and can do gymnastics out of the water that would put Cirque du Soleil to shame. All powered by that fluke/tail. And that fluke is a flirting mechanism—but that is so second chakra!!

Our feathered friends have a light skeletal system, obviously necessary to take flight. They have a high metabolic rate and oxygen supply. Their bones seem hollow (not all), their beak makes up for the lack of teeth—they were made for flight! Birds have (free) caudal vertebrae, and the end of their tail is a triangular plate formed of the fused caudal vertebrae, what is known as the pygostyle. The flattened mass of bones and tissue surrounding it is the anchor for the tail muscles and feathers. The tail feathers of each species are specific to their needs. For example, penguins, puffins, and boobies are going to have an old-school long and straight pygostyle to dive underwater, powered by that first chakra tail! Whereas the pygostyle in a raptor has to support a lot more feathers for flight and navigation midair.

Meridians and Traditional Chinese Medicine

In Traditional Chinese Medicine (TCM), several of the meridians start somewhere in the root chakra. A meridian is a pathway where energy flows. Each meridian is associated with an organ system, and that organ system is associated with an emotion. TCM is a whole approach to health and well-being.

The Conception Vessel (CV) meridian starts at the root chakra and runs up the front of the body, like a zipper in a meridian suit. It stores and facilitates the flow of energy for things like injuries or deficient organs. Known as the Sea of Yin, it runs up the front like a fountain, feeding the first to fifth chakras.

The Governing Vessel (GV) meridian starts at the root in the back and flows up the back, over the crown and down to the roof of the mouth. This is called creating the microcosmic orbit. It is a stronger energy known as the Sea of Yang.

Several meridians start on the hind feet: liver, kidney, and spleen.

Several meridians end on the hind feet: gallbladder, urinary bladder, and stomach.

Excerpted from my second book, *Energy Healing for Animals* (Sounds True, 2015):

- The gallbladder (yang) meridian starts on the hind legs, travels up the outside of the leg and up to the torso and on either side of the lower part of the left hind leg, and follows up the shoulder and neck, making quite a squiggly trail between the eyes and the ears.
- The Conception Vessel (yin) starts right under the tail and moves up the midline on the belly to the top of the bottom lip. It is not associated with an organ.
- The Governing Vessel (yang) starts right under the tail, comes up over the back up to the head, and ends between the nose and the top of the mouth of the animal. It is not associated with an organ, yet it is connected to and with all of the yang organs and meridians.
- The kidney meridian (yin) starts at the main pad of the hind paws, follows up the inside of the hind legs, and trails up the belly and to the chest. It parallels the Conception Vessel.
- The bladder or urinary meridian (yang) begins at the inside of the eyes on both sides, parallel with the Governing Vessel. It then follows down the back and down the hind quarters and ends on the outside toe. If you only learn about one meridian, the bladder meridian is the fascinating one to study, as it contains associated points for all of the organs. These can not only help in healing but also indicate where there is an imbalance in general, or an imbalance associated with a particular organ. More on this in Part Two.

TCM physical activities related to the meridians in the feet:

- Arteries
- Veins
- Flow in life
- Blood flow
- Circulation
- Immune
- Challenges

Putting It All Together: Survive or Thrive?

Whether human or animal, the body is this amazing complex structure that is built to heal and adjust itself in any given circumstance. Homeostasis is the regulation of temperature, equilibrium between elements, and balance of physiological duties. When in trouble, or too much of an imbalance, homeostasis can be the body's response to fighting to stay alive. Any physiological, mental, emotional, or environmental stress is always nipping at our potential for balanced, perfect health. Some first chakra health challenges:

- **Immune-compromised**

The immune system is the body's defense against illness, infection, virus, or bacteria. Parasites play a big role in this, they are not necessarily recognized in Western medicine, but many doctors of acupuncture or chiropractic see parasites as an underlying cause that can weaken the immune system. Candida can also weaken the immune system. The lymph system plays an active role in the cleanup of our system, it is the underground sewage system that removes all fluids that leak out of the blood vessels.

- **Overly active immune system, like allergic reactions**

The overly active system can respond to the environment, dust, smoke, chemicals in the household and have an allergic reaction, which can be expressed through the nasal passages, the lungs and/or the skin.

- **Autoimmune disorders**

Autoimmune disorders are where the body attacks the healthy cells and tissues. Some examples of this are: diabetes, lupus, and rheumatoid arthritis.

- **Ongoing gut issues because of a lot of medication due to often life-threatening disease as a baby**

This is more common than people even realize. The amount of antibiotics or chemical wormers that go into saving an animal's life often creates a compromised immune system because of the weakened gut. Thousands and thousands of animal medical intuition scans later, often this gut needs repair from the original survival mechanism of medication.

- **Degenerative Diseases**

Degenerative diseases also fall under the first chakra. They usually lead to disability and/or death. For animals who feel they must mask, they can become reactive or internalize, and this can also be covered by the emotional/energetic component of the first chakra.

- **Recurring injuries or injuries that happened as a baby**

Often injuries fall under the first chakra, particularly if they are in the hind end, or are recurring. It will threaten their emotional safety, even if they "mask" as easy going. If the injury is big enough, keeping them mobile would require a fair amount of care.

- **Birth defects or immunocompromised babies**

Of course, animals that were born with defects and/or health challenges fall under a first chakra challenge. The animal's experience from day one would likely seem like a fight for survival and then they would need special care throughout their lifetime.

- **Lameness**

Lameness puts any animal on hyperawareness. They become protective of the lame limb. As a result of their vigilance and protection of the injured limb, they can have an additional injury occur on the corresponding bilateral limb. In the wild, lameness often equals death.

The reason many of these things fall under the first chakra is because, if they were in the wild, they wouldn't survive. There isn't an insulin booth in the forest for those diabetic bobcats. There isn't wound care for a wolf. Maybe there are pigeons with allergies. But they don't last long. Any of the above-mentioned challenges would equal "game over" in the wild.

There is no little squirrel nurse tending to the wound of an injured bear or a postoperative peregrine falcon. Although, I do love that image. That is why many of these things fall under the first chakra. In fact, if wildlife is sent to a rehab center due to an injury or life-threatening event, the whole question becomes whether they can survive back out in the wild.

Even the smallest virus in a housecat, early onset hip dysplasia in a dog, or a life-threatening infection in a horse can change the animal's behavior—react or internalize—, can shift dynamics with the other animals in the household, and possibly inform the trajectory of that personality throughout that animal's lifetime. You can take the sweetest cat in the world, come at it with enough medication and suddenly you need the kind of gloves that protect you from hawk talons, protective headgear, and a Michelin man suit to keep from being slashed to death.

Students love to say, "This animal has a blocked first chakra." I always ask them, "Oh, are they dying? Are they unable to poop?" Because to me, the dynamics of the emotional and energetic can be advised by the physical reality. And vice versa. The physical reality of an animal can be created by the emotional and energetic environment. Caroline Myss says, "The biography becomes the biology."

But the truth is, nothing is blocked. Perhaps it lacks energy. Or needs a little juice. But if a chakra is blocked you truly need an ambulance, not an energy healer.

First Chakra Emotions and Energetics

Red is the color associated with this chakra. Vibrant red. Red hot excitement, enthusiasm, or passion. This energy can also be red hot anger, furious, frustration, and reactive. These animals can often redirect their anger, passion, or frustration on the wrong being, that is whoever is right in front of them.

For humans, the first chakra represents the tribe and family, the family of origin as well as the family we have created to provide safety. It represents our culture, our country of origin, our companions, our friends, the organizations we relate to, and workmates. As we evolve, it includes the chosen tribes of people we connect to along our personal journey of growth. Or it is the people we stay wounded with. It is our life force, it is home. The first chakra is safety to its core, and our sense of well-being.

In many ways, to have a first chakra experience is to step away from these tribes in our youth and establish ourselves. It is also about coming back as we care for our parents in their end of life. A first chakra viewpoint would be looking through the lens of safety. We always use that filter to feel into our safety and security in any given situation or group gathering. For humans, the first chakra is also about our home—internally and physically—literally, our home, and safety.

Because the first chakra is all about our safety and security, it represents being grounded on Planet Earth and making sound decisions. Conversely, it could be about how our wounding took over and created an environment for us until we became conscious enough to evolve out of that. Someone with early wounding or past life first chakra trauma may spend their lifetime mildly or overly suspicious, looking over their shoulder, not trusting, and may be prone to joining cults.

For animals, the first chakra represents their pack, herd, colony, flock, pride of origin, and then the multispecies family that they have been adopted into. First chakra experiences include their relationships with other animals of the same species. Of course, it is also all about how they get along with other animals of other species—in or out of their home. This also relates to their "positioning" in the home. Are they the dominant one? Timid? The first chakra experience involves how much they value the physical home they live in as well as the simple experiences, like riding in the car, going on a walk, or meeting someone new—human or otherwise.

Not to mention how they view things like going to the veterinarian. A simple nail trim and a blood test can turn into a Friday the Thirteenth horror movie sequel.

Unless it is an embedded, limbic trauma, animals can evolve out of their wounding. They live in the moment, so sometimes it can be done on their own through time. They can also truly heal and settle with great guardians and guidance. Sometimes our contract as the human is to create such a safe space that they can have all of their freak-out moments with us buffering it until they say "okay, life is good!" Sometimes we spend a lifetime managing their old wounding as it prevails in a current pattern.

Two Legs and a Head

I always say when an animal goes into fear, it becomes two legs and a head. This is when the head goes up, the hind end comes down. The amygdala, a small organ in the middle of the brain, alerts the entire system. Stress hormones, cortisol and adrenaline, are released, the heart rate increases, and blood flows into the limbs. It's as if they leave their body and function from the shoulders forward, and they are not thinking. A horse will swing its butt around as if it isn't even attached. Dogs drop their hind end and tuck their tails. And cats become hovercrafts. When an animal is on alert a lot, I always say that the neck and throat develop the periscope muscle! Their forelegs become a powerful force of nature.

You can see this phenomenon out in nature, the head lifts on high alert and the entire herd is off! In our homes, we can prepare for things like leash reactivity or a spooky horse. We will see the ears forward and the gaze fixate. Often you will see your dog's hind end lower, and then launch.

In the wild, the animals have an opportunity to release this adrenaline as they continue to run or fly after the threat is gone. In our homes, unless they have a great exercise routine, that stress builds up in their system without an outlet. So, the two legs and a head experiences become their release of this pent-up sensation.

First Chakra Behavior, Dynamics, and Relationships

The first chakra is all about security and safety for animals. Their behavior would reflect that through fight, flight, or freeze. This chakra includes all their senses on guard. This is a hind end that is amped and ready to activate into flight or launch. The flip side of that would be seeing a very grounded animal and how well this animal is listening to and connected with their human counterpart and the other animals in their multispecies home.

An animal's understanding of the perimeters in life is usually based on pushing up against boundaries to discover where exactly they stand. For example, male elephants aged 12 to 15 will leave the herd and create a band of boys. They are likely kicked out because of their juvenile shenanigans. And puberty. We see this in herds of horses as well. We don't see this (puberty driven dismissal) in our homes because of the spay and neuter practices we uphold in the US. We don't experience the individuation that is the result of active hormones. We don't see: "You must leave!" Nor do we experience the matriarch societies that many species develop.

Yet, we see our animals push up against each other when they are young or new to the household. Often, an animal will play nice for the first six months of being adopted and then see how far they can go once they feel a little settled. Once they have pushed up enough, the ruling forces, the environment itself, other animals, and/or the human would push back, and the individual would know where it stands and who they are.

No other species greets with a handshake and looks eye to eye. Most species dance around each other's butts! They sneak a smell in, determining their own safety based on pheromones released from their new potential friend. Pheromones are chemical signals that create a profile of who that animal is by scent. This scent profile can help someone—the smeller—determine territory, sexuality, social status, and bonding. In other words, butt smelling, usually of the same species, cuts right to the chase.

Multispecies living doesn't have the science behind it but based on how quickly my dogs get their not-so-sneaky noses in my cat's butt, information is being given out between species as well.

While we're talking about butts, let's talk about tails because they tell a tale! Tails will alert us as to how animals are feeling with some subtle, and some not-so-subtle, physical attributes.

Sometimes the tucked tail is a signal for someone else in the pack to take over. The tail can set up a boundary quickly. The tail tucked is a way of pulling their energy in and getting a feel for the whole ecosystem.

And some animals, with eyes on the sides of their head like horses, birds, cetaceans, and more, have the ability to see behind them. Their sight is such that they are seeing each side independently, yet together. They have blind spots directly in front of them and directly behind them. Yet, their sight allows for them to see most of what is behind them.

Animals are masters of masking. Hiding pain was built into their DNA ages ago to protect themselves from predators while they are sick or injured. They may not let on that they aren't as settled when they first move into a household. As I have mentioned before, after years and years of watching animals enter new homes, and acting as if they fit like a glove, I am convinced that they audition for at least six months. After that, the real personality comes out. Sometimes it is not always the dog or cat the people picked! Masking is definitely a survival behavior.

Animals will recognize their likeness. I've seen border collies meet other border collies at the beach and, upon meeting, feel compelled to competitively round up all the Golden Retrievers. When I lived in the Seattle area, I was high on a hill above a flood zone. I always let this woman who lived down in the valley evacuate her horses to my farm. My horse Gabrielle is an Arabian who had always lived in barns with big warmbloods and thoroughbreds before I started living with my horses. When the woman from the valley evacuated her Arabians up to my farm, Gabrielle would let out a primal scream that translated to something like, "My people!"

Some of our household animal companions like safety in numbers, meaning the more the better. Some want to keep the household exclusive. And others like to fly solo. In Chapter 10 we will run through ideas to shift your household chakra by chakra. In the meantime, if you are having relationship issues between yourself and an animal, your household is experiencing challenges between animals, or a recent dynamic appeared, here are some good questions to ponder as you read through some of the stories of the first chakra in action:

1. Is my own world safe and secure? What adjustments do I have to make to provide that for my animals?
2. Is the chaos of my childhood so familiar, I have recreated it in my adult life and am subjecting my animals to what I grew up in?
3. This is not my first chakra "survival" experience, it is theirs. How am I supporting their experience?
4. Has my animal ever known safety?
5. Is my animal able to self-soothe?
6. Am I providing safety for them?

Stories

Delilah

I share this story in *Emotional Freedom Technique for Animals* (Findhorn Press, 2023) but it is worth telling it again:

Delilah is my own dog who suffered from "leash exuberance" with a sudden onset at age four. When we were off the property, she would be so excited when she saw another dog in the distance, then in a split second, she was suddenly reactive. It seemed to come out of nowhere. And I mean scary-seeming reactive.

Delilah is a border collie cross, Sagittarius party girl who was raised in part by me and two older dog siblings. Olivia (one-half border collie, one-quarter German shepherd, one-quarter rottweiler, 100 percent Scorpio) was about ten when Delilah was adopted, and Isabella (Supermodel black lab, Libra) was roughly six. They all played hard, worked hard, and loved hard. Weekly, we would go on a large pack walk with a dog trainer. Sometimes up to seventeen dogs including my three. Each week, Delilah was introduced to several new dogs and the old standbys.

When Delilah was about four years old, we moved to California, and within a year, we lost both Olivia and Isabella. And we adopted Abby (black lab/shar-pei, Libra) between those two losses. While we had some dog friends here and there, we weren't in large packs anymore.

One day, I took my dogs to the beach. When I got out of the car, I had to put my dogs on leashes. As we walked the trail to get to the beach, Delilah was getting more and more excited. She loved the beach. But then, to my shock, as we passed dogs, Delilah became unglued, barking and raging at the other dogs. She went from zero to sixty in a nano-second. It took every ounce of my strength to keep Delilah with me. And I handle horses daily.

Meanwhile, Abby was unphased.

I chalked it up to the fact that we hadn't been to the beach since Isabella died, and Delilah was excited. But it kept happening. I had to gear up to go anywhere. I was in shock. And sad for the happy dog Delilah usually was in the company of others.

As I worked with a trainer and did Emotional Freedom Technique (EFT) Tapping, it came together for me. Essentially, I had allowed Olivia and Isabella to raise Delilah. While neither elder was ever reactive, they were protective of our old farm. Here I am, the one who talks about Emotional Leadership in both of my previous books, and now with Delilah, I was not the emotional leader.

I needed some training!! Without that leadership, Delilah was confused, scared, and honestly, didn't know how to be.

I am happy to say, between the tapping, training, and me stepping in as the emotional leader, we can pass just about any situation without her giving it a second thought. If I see her assuming the position of blast off into reactivity, I simply say "leave it." And she does.

Ella

Ella wouldn't know how to be "off duty" if you paid her in dog bones for the rest of her life. A German shepherd cross meant that duty was her middle name. She thrived in the household with her littermate brother, Gunner, Addie—a younger bloodhound who worshiped Ella, and Buddy, a fierce min pin who would love to take over Ella's jobs and authority. Ella also lived with a hedgehog, six cats, two adult humans, Sarah and Ben, and four boys under the age of ten. The property of her home butted up against open space where wild pigs, deer, and all of Florida's wildlife flourished. It was a lot to manage. But Ella loved every ounce of it, chaos and all.

As Ella was getting older, her path to the back door to bark at wild pigs might be littered with other dogs and cats and her hips were quite weak. When everyone was home, she was manager deluxe. But unfortunately, a couple of times, it was caught on home surveillance cameras that Ella had gone after Addie. One of those times involved hospitalization and life-threatening injuries.

As "duty first," frustration and masked pain were hitting a crescendo. Ella's pent-up energy blasted like an ancient volcano onto Addie and unfortunately it was blood, rather than lava, flowing. There was no lack of love, it was a true pain-masking-frustration redirect. Until the humans heard from the students in my advanced class just how painful those hips were, Sarah and Ben didn't realize how much Ella was masking the pain. In the wild, Ella may have gone after someone young but then she would eventually be ousted as she would have made the pack weak. Hind end pain creates a bigger threat to survival for a duty-filled girl.

Thankfully, Ben and Sarah are getting the training, the EFT healing they need, and are managing the situation through crates when they are not home. Thankfully for Ella, she has the most loving, understanding humans around.

Winter

Winter, a beautiful Bernese Mountain dog, was introduced to me via his person Ruth, as she was challenged by his fear of pulling a cart. The first of many animal communication and healing sessions with all of her animals over the years was initiated by this challenge. Ruth enjoys things to the fullest capacity. She had another dog at the time named Max, who was winning titles left and right in obedience and carting. In their time off, she and her husband would take the dogs up to their mountain cabin and they had a very vigorous outdoor life hiking, snowshoeing, and cross-country skiing.

Meanwhile, back in the city, Winter and Max were the darlings of the neighborhood as Max carted Ruth to work from her home to her office down on Lake Union in Seattle with Winter by his side. However, in the show ring, Winter exhibited disdain and fear at the idea of pulling the cart. The idea that Winter was afraid of the cart was challenging for Ruth for a number of reasons: Ruth loved to show her dogs; Ruth enjoyed her ride to work; Ruth doesn't really fail!

Somewhere in Ruth was a disappointment that could have become consuming. When I connected with Winter, he showed me a picture of some sort of tarp or tent or something coming down on him and scaring him. All of the apparatus that was involved with the cart reminded him of this scary experience and for him, all he wanted to do was get away or just shut down.

Once Ruth heard this, she had something to work with. She began desensitizing him to the cart and continued to get him to engage positively. Eventually Ruth and Winter were back in the show ring, and he won his titles. But she redirected his energy to show him doing things he loved. She gave up on the cart as something he had to continue with.

Many years later, the true glory of that communication session and Ruth's assertive approach paid off in ways that fall into the *extraordinary* category. Winter was diagnosed with Degenerative Myelopathy, a disease that affects the spinal cord in many breeds. It is chronic and progressive, resulting in paralysis.

Winter, once he lost the use of his legs, not only took to the wheels that were offered to him like a champ, but it's also as if his entire life, he was born to be the ambassador to humans skeptical about wheels. He took to it with the zest that Ruth and her husband go to their mountain home and soak in and experience every ounce of mountain life around them.

There was no stopping Winter. He experienced freedom and was able to go back to the things he loved. Getting down to the river, trudging through the river rocks, being on the hikes, meadows, shores, and even hiking up to a high mountain lake—all that he had enjoyed with four good legs was now available to him again. He also went back on ski trails and even herded.

Toward the end of his life, Winter allowed his brother Tonka to pull him in a four-wheel cart, in other words, none of his legs worked well. He was experiencing fatigue in the front end due to compensation because the hind end didn't work at all. This was a true healing as he was competitive with Tonka for Ruth's love. This is also a true first chakra triumph story. First there was his blinding fear (first chakra), and a simple animal communication made his underlying terror clear to Ruth. She took action, had patience and persistence, and then—ultimately—when he lost the use on his hind end (first chakra), the cart, the wheels, the apparatus, and Ruth's ride saved the day.

Speaking of first chakra triumph, the flip side of surviving is thriving. There are plenty of animals—and people—who experience life-threatening situations and come out better than before the circumstance. There are animals—I've had plenty of them—who have had just brutal starts in life but if attention isn't drawn there, they thrive. This is because they are in the moment and brand-new and fabulous moments are presented to them. There are animals—and people—who seem to have the karma of "I'm fine, someone will take care of this, now hand me my squeaky toy!"

Let's keep each other safe.

THE SECOND CHAKRA—EXCHANGE OF ENERGY

"Our consciousness moves from a feeling of unity to the realization of difference. Our understanding of self now includes an awareness of the other. Connecting with another, desire arises, and with it our emotions and sexuality. We long to unite, to overcome our separateness, to reach out and grow. These are all aspects of consciousness at the second chakra—all of which induce change."

—Anodea Judith, Ph.D., *Wheels of Life: A User's Guide to the Chakra System*

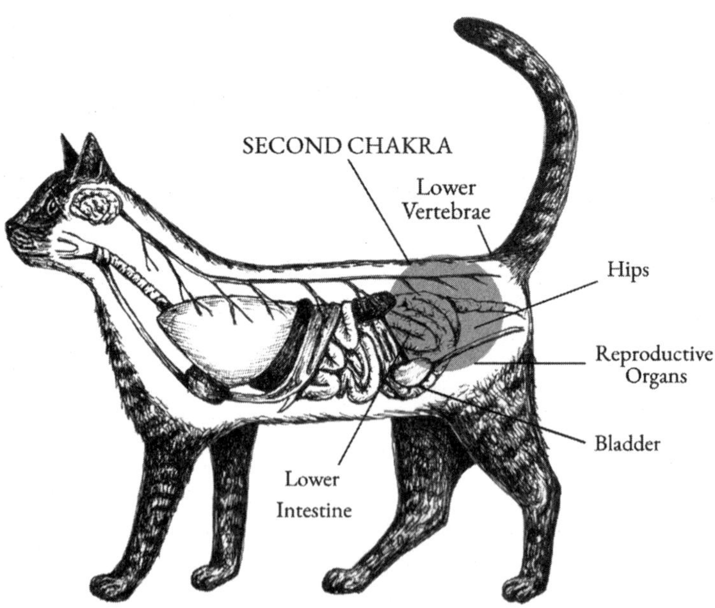

Fig. 3: The second chakra (sacral chakra)

Dolphins—The Joy of Playfulness

I have had the pleasure of swimming with wild dolphins. I was lucky to experience the same pods of bottlenose and Atlantic spotted dolphins, for two weeks out of the year for seven years. And for seven years, I took people on these dolphin trips. I would love to think that the dolphins recognized me as I recognized them from birthmarks and scars. Let's just say I know I was a familiar, admiring energy for them.

Unless you are a regular underwater visitor, my description will fall flat of what it is like to be in their world. Imagine slipping into a kaleidoscope, the optical instrument that reflects two or more surfaces (mirrors), only you are one of the mirrors reflecting to the other mirror. The dolphins are the other mirror and what is being reflected back and forth in this instrument now is a celebration of joy, love, beauty, sensuousness, and more. And it is in the bluest, most intoxicatingly beautiful water. These gorgeous beings swimming near you are as curious about you as you are about them. It is breathtaking.

These dolphins knew the boat and would come play in the wake, like little kids, catching the free ride from the white waters the boat produced. When we would stop, they would often play under the boat, and pop out on the other side, and fly into the air as if to entertain us. We would all chorus "OOOooohhhhhh." Someone would have to be in an aluminum suit to block the telepathic messages of love being sent to them by the dolphins. Yet, those dolphins aren't doing a thing for us, they are doing it for themselves. They are simply embodying the playful nature we know that dolphins display.

And to slip into the water with them is a whole other experience. They continue in their delight and speed. Their bodies are solid, fluid, and graceful. Their seraphic faces with their beatific smile leads one to believe that they were dropped straight from the heavens. They swim by and assess your whole being with their inquisitive eye.

That curiosity, that joyful playfulness, and that alleged smile have gotten them into trouble with humans. We have taken that "smile" and exploited it as we've associated it with a certain relationship to us. Or worse, *for* us. Dolphins are used in entertainment, kept in pools which would be like putting your kids in something the size of a bathtub and expecting them to grow and live out their days. Bottlenose dolphins, in particular, have been plucked from the sea for our entertainment. They have better flexibility because they have fewer fused vertebrae in their necks than other dolphins. When they turn and look at us, it is human-like, and we recognize them to be like us.

Therefore, people have believed the marketing about Sea World and other aquariums that dolphins are smiling while they are working. Well, they are no more smiling than orangutans are lonely and wistful—nor are cheetahs crying. These are anatomical features and structures of their faces. These built-in features aren't displaying any emotion whatsoever. In fact, we know the dolphins in performance situations experience extreme anxiety and will wear their teeth down on the cement, they will neurotically swim in circles and much, much worse.

Yet swimming with them in the wild where they display their natural curiosity over shiny objects like camera lenses and what we are wearing brings on a certain energetic smile for us humans. "Of all the things they could be doing in the vast ocean, and they are picking to play with us," gets expressed at some point by every human on those dolphin trips. The truth is, as I dry off after being in the ocean with them, I also have those kinds of thoughts, and that sentiment makes each and every cell in my body smile.

Dolphins seem to also have an energetic smile with each other. One thing can be said for dolphins in the wild, they are in full agency of themselves as individuals. The second chakra is all about developing relationships, sexuality, and a lot more that we will discuss in this chapter. But we can see the intoxication of the second chakra when we're underwater long enough and witness dolphin orgies. Yes, orgies.

Dolphins will do a drive-by masturbation like you might hand off a latte to a friend. I have had times underwater when I would see the juveniles were off doing juvenile things like diving deep and seemingly in formation and then they would come back up to surface mouthing and biting each other in just the way my dogs play under my desk when I'm trying to teach. But the rest of the pod? The adults? It was full on, full pod, fully engaged in a swinging multi-partnered dolphin sex party.

So, if a dolphin is actually smiling, perhaps we know why. It wasn't a rape culture like roosters or other animals. It is joy in their entire being, including their sexuality. Everyone got attention, young, old, male, and female. It is a true celebration of embodying their beingness. I would watch Atlantic spotted dolphins breeze in among the bottlenose and you would think that some exotic celebrity had just swam in. All the attention would go to them for a moment, and it would feel as though the paparazzi were there flashing cameras. For a while I thought I wanted to come back in my next life as an Atlantic spotted dolphin. But then I went through menopause and let go of that.

Dolphins experience a freedom in the wild that we will never know. Probably not in our lifetime, in this incarnation anyway. If any one of those female dolphins were in our high school class our collective culture would take over and we would all simultaneously call her a slut, when perhaps we were secretly envious of her freedom. We might also loudly promote the fact that she lacked morals and had a loose character.

The sexuality that they enjoy is something that we as humans don't experience. Even in periods of history when sexual freedom bursts through the door, it is as if it pushes up against the moral boundary and rarely has a lasting effect. In fact, usually the pendulum swings back to some sort of puritan way of being and it's talked about with scorn under hushed tones. Others would continue, negating any restrictions and be considered amoral. More second chakra shame for humans.

Dolphins aren't the only wild ones in the animal kingdom. Bonobo monkeys are famous for "make love, not war." As a result of their activity, they do have strong social bonds and resolve conflict easily, unlike their dramatic cousins, chimpanzees. Certain birds, lizards, flies, lions, frogs, and walruses (who knew) are not monogamous and know how to party. I've spent time with several wild herds of horses, and sex just casually happens within minutes and then they carry on grazing as if nothing happened.

Second Chakra Symbolism

The second chakra represents a seemingly broad, yet focused, spectrum. It symbolizes the vital life force, creativity, pleasure, self-expression, intimacy, connection, relationships—particularly one-on-one relationships, the ones we seek beyond the primary relationships, sex, and money. It is represented by the lotus flower which represents the cycle of birth, death, and rebirth. The second chakra is freedom, flow, and fluidity. The ability to receive and serve all in one fell swoop!

Personal power and agency over oneself are aspects of the second Chakra. This means understanding one's self-worth and finding value in it.

And did I mention sex? Oh yeah, I think we covered that with the dolphin stories. The second chakra is also about fertility, and is where the spark of creativity is born. And this is juicy creativity, inspirational creativity, creativity that was just simply downloaded, born, or birthed. It is the kind of creativity that can come to you in one moment and then seem to cook in the oven of the second chakra for a long time. The kind of idea that won't go away.

The womb is physically here. The amniotic fluid lives here. The second chakra is all about procreation, birthing, nurturance, tenderness, desire, and pleasure.

Some say this is the home of the divine feminine.

The color is orange. The element of the second chakra is water. Still waters run deep, emotions live here. Deep family histories, deep scars, and wounds. This is the very place where the deep, buried secrets live. Money and the exchange of energy lives here. Some people see money as power. Some see their own self-worth in terms of monetary value here. The second chakra is where money and power become interchangeable.

The shadow side of the second chakra can be the challenging feelings that come with money and sex—guilt, control, and the need for power. It also loves the blame and shame game.

What does all this symbolism mean for the animals? What is money for an animal? Where is their power in all of this? Unfortunately, for the animals, this is where the deepest, dirtiest secrets of the animal kingdom reside. And not because they are having repressed thoughts about themselves. Rather, the real truth is that the second chakra is all about exchange. It can be the exchange of bodily fluids, it can be the exchange of currency, it can be the exchange of affection. But sadly, in this case, much of our human buried secrets is an uneven exchange. Our continued exploitation of animals throughout history is a shared, second-chakra to second-chakra secret that deserves unearthing. This is where sex, money, and power are intermingled in a most disturbing way with the animal kingdom. And the animals are always on the wrong side of that. Symbolically we often see that animals suffer from the Stockholm Syndrome, where they admire their captor.

Certainly, animals find their power within their pack, pride, or family system. They have hierarchies and positions and sometimes they fight for power. The more spoiled the animal is, the more they know their power over us.

We aren't geared toward empowering them. In fact, even using the word "pet," which means an animal that is kept as a companion, has some detractors. I personally like to use the words "animal companion" or simply "family" and I definitely veer from the word "owner" and replace it with "guardian." PETA says that the word "pet" is patronizing. I would say the word "pet" has a "less than" quality to it. And the "ownership" of animals doesn't provide full agency for them, even if we are the guardian who keeps them safe. I always say I want my animals well-adjusted enough so that if something happened to me, they would be sad, but they would bounce back with a soft landing.

For many domesticated animals, the "power" of the second chakra gets lost. In other words, there is an expiration date for their "power" and often the expiration date includes eviction. Too many shelters fill up with older animals. Many people "rehome" their animals once they have served their purpose. They are sent off to pasture. A pasture would be an improvement. They are sent to live their days in a cement cell. Horses are "retired."

As long as animals are legal property, there is a certain "value" we put on them and it is nothing short of enslavement. We might look at their bloodlines to find value or look at the bill of sale to see their monetary value. Yet, an animal may see their own value during an animal communication session as "I have a big heart," "I'm a pleaser," "I'm a great protector even if my hearing is going, my bark is fierce," "I'm a teacher," or

"I am a solid friend." Unfortunately, in a court of law, the value would get tipped on the scales toward the monetary.

When we are exchanging big money for animals, they are commodities, they are things, and no matter how good a home we give them, many could be said to be enslaved.

Of course, people will buy animals. This isn't going to stop today. Breeders are going to continue to breed. People are going to continue to want purebred animals. But this whole world could be reformed. Again, I don't have the answers, I'm just opening a conversation about one of the many second chakra shadow aspects of the animal kingdom.

Second Chakra Species-Specific/Breed-Specific

The second chakra is all about buried secrets. At the end of the day, the only difference between your French Bulldog and the pig down the street or the cow on slaughter row, is that your French Bulldog is lucky. But they were all bred for our benefit.

Domestication

We can't forget the sexual aspect of the second chakra. Sexuality is free for animals, except our domesticated friends. Pet overpopulation is a very disturbing reality as it ends up as a genocide on animals in the shelter system here in the US. Spaying and castrating—neutering female and male animals respectively—is necessary in our current conditions.

Unwanted pets—among many other forms of suffering that animals experience—are a large part of the deep shadow of this second chakra for animals. While some animals experience their full sexuality, dogs and cats are living with our inability to take responsibility, our carelessness as a species and ultimately, our inexhaustible consumerism.

The Shadow Side of the Second Chakra

There is another cost to our convenience. Ovaries and testes, both known as gonads—the female and male reproduction organs—are also considered to be endocrine glands. The way in which animals are desexed means that as the organs/glands are removed, so is all the tissue. If the animal is young, the endocrine, glandular, and hormonal systems have not fully developed.

Estrogen plays a big role in skeletal maturation, bone growth, and development. When estrogen is not produced, an imbalance is created that can lead to growth plates remaining open, which leads to joint issues; there is a higher rupture rate in bone—not to mention, hip dysplasia, bone cancer, and more.

This leads to other endocrine issues like adrenal disease, Cushing's disease, hypothyroidism, and other irreversible metabolic diseases.

Dr. Karen Becker is leading the charge on helping people to understand sterilization vs. desexing and how this spares their parts, meaning that the ovaries and testes would be better serving our animal friends, their long-term health and even their longevity. This would be a modified spay for females, and a vasectomy versus castrating for males. This would also mean that there would have to be a total revamp in the shelter system, and the smaller rescue world.

This is obviously a much bigger conversation that deserves its own topic, perhaps even its own bookshelf or library. In order to revamp shelters to create more long-term health for our animal friends, that would require a lot more human duty, education, trust, training skills, accountability, and a whole lot more responsibility from individual adopters. And that may not happen anytime soon.

I'm sure there are people in Europe who are reading this book and are astonished at our situation. They have free roaming dogs who are on voice command. Their females are kept inside during their heat.

It appears, felines don't have the same health issues. Or the research isn't there yet. As we all know, cats still rule parts of the Middle East. There is a wonderful documentary called Kedi, about cats ruling and roaming the streets of Istanbul. When I was teaching in Beijing, China, cats were so beloved in the small alleyways that were lined with gorgeous traditional shops. They are not about to go neuter or spay these cats in these cultures, rather they co-exist in a way that Americans certainly cannot fathom. The humans in many of these communities accept, welcome, and feed—literally and figuratively—these territories.

And nobody is doing anything in the horse world but promoting early castration of horses, somewhat understandably. In the case of horses, the aggression of a stallion is not for the faint of heart.

There is a reason that things like cars are associated with horsepower. One thousand pounds of massive muscle coming right at you at 20 mph is a sight to behold and a threat to your life. I would find clearance, a bush, a different path, anything to get out of the way of that force of nature! Before I enter a pen with a stallion to do animal communication, EFT, or anything other healing modality, no matter how sweet they are, I know where my exits are. I'm usually called for an aggression issue.

Ninety-five percent of the time, horse people who do have stallions have a healthy respect for what this requires. It is the ultimate combination of what I talk about in all of my books—animal communication, energy healing, training, holistic care, and management. In other words, every bit of their life, their safety, the safety of others is thought through completely by the human. Emotional leadership at its best.

Like I said, I have no answer, just questions and points to bring to the table. Sadly, for over thirty years, I get called by shelters and rescues to help the "unadoptable" animals because of our throwaway society. There are millions of animals a year that were never given a voice, they were euthanized because the shelter had to make more room for the "adoptable" animals coming in.

Second Chakra Organs, Systems, Structure, and Meridians

The second chakra is orange. Physically, it is all about reproduction. It is also about holding energetic space for and cooking that inspired idea. For humans, the second chakra is located between the belly button and the pubic bone. To find the second chakra on animals, we look on the top of the animal in the region of the lower back, hips, and sacrum. It also goes straight through to their belly or teats. This is the area that is visible, available, and vulnerable to the world.

Organs and Systems

Physically, the second chakra governs all of our reproductive organs, the bladder, hips, lower vertebrae, sacrum, lower intestine, and the pelvic shield for all of these organs. The cecum on the right side of the lower abdomen feeds into the colon and more second chakra activity takes place in the lower colon, leading to the rectum. The second chakra includes the female organs and hormonal glands, the teats, as well as the male sexual organs.

- Physiological systems at work here: reproductive (produce BABIES!).
- Endocrine systems at work here: ovaries.

- Nerve plexus: sacral hypogastric plexus (speaks to the pelvic and perineal organs), Peripheral Nervous System (PNS).
- Spine: sacral/sacrum, S1 – S5, that affect nerve communication to the lower portion of the body.

Meridians and Traditional Chinese Medicine

The meridians that run through the second chakra are the Governing Vessel (GV), Conception Vessel (CV), Bladder (BL), Stomach (St), Gallbladder (GB), Spleen/Pancreas (Sp), Kidney (Ki), and Liver (Liv).

In Traditional Chinese Medicine, the bladder is related to shock. The bladder's sister meridian, the kidney, is associated with fear.

Putting It All Together: Exchange and Elimination

The second chakra is also the process center for exchange and elimination. If we look at all the organs and systems here, it is built to connect, express, receive, release, and eliminate. If any of that is out of balance—emotionally or energetically—physical challenges may arise.

Some of the challenges here are infertility, impotence, lower back pain, urinary challenges, and diseases of the reproductive organs. For humans, this is entangled with sexual shame. As we've been discussing, animals know nothing about this!

Upon returning from a big animal communication and energy healing workshop I taught in Steamboat, Colorado, one of the students reached out to me and shared that she didn't want to say anything in front of anyone, but she was unable to get pregnant, no matter how often she and her husband tried! It had been a couple of years. I suggested that she work on that second chakra, to put a lot of attention there and do the clearing I had just taught. She was pregnant weeks later! I have an incredible fourth-chakra follow-up and an 18 years' later story to this.

Many large dog breeds start to lose their hind end in this area. As activity dwindles, the relationship changes. Dogs who have chased the kids around the neighborhood in family fun, have also watched “their” kids go off to college or become adults. As their wards leave the nest, they now lie quietly in the family room, and have earned this downtime. The dynamics between animals shift as the elder slows down.

Horses get a little hitch in their giddyup here. They aren’t as easily striking off with that hind leg to pick up the correct “lead” in front. The hips and sacrum are easily overlooked as to why a horse isn’t “performing” as they once did.

We see cats not leaping through the trees as much when this area breaks down in the aging process. We also see litter box challenges because the hips are so tight, and cats are the masters of masking pain. They can’t get in and out of the litter box like they used to. People don’t pick up on it because the cat is acting fine. Then litter box issues appear to be a “behavioral issue” when, in truth, it could very well be the hind end.

Litter box issues usually have many physical reasons behind it. If nothing else, the muscle memory of a painful infection. Interstitial, or idiopathic cystitis, is bladder pain with an unknown cause. The symptoms include the need to urinate right away. Sadly, I think that this is why the shelters in the US are full of “unadoptable cats.” Humans can at least express this discomfort. Cats’—and dogs’—only expression is to urinate.

More typical animal issues, excerpted from my book *Emotional Freedom Technique for Animals and their Humans*:

"Urinary Tract Infections (UTI's) are a leading cause for inappropriate peeing, as is kidney and/or bladder disease. These are easily diagnosed, but two conditions that are exceptionally painful and don't get diagnosed easily are idiopathic cystitis (which can lead to crystals and a clogging of the urethra that could result in a major surgery, if not death) and osteoarthritis/joint pain.

Idiopathic cystitis is a swelling of the bladder wall or urethra. If it goes undiagnosed for a long time, it leads to a thickening of the bladder wall. Having done animal medical intuition on thousands of animals with this condition, it is very painful and comes on quickly, feeling like an ongoing emergency in the body. Sadly, this gets overlooked until it is a medical emergency. Any sort of pressure emotionally would feel like pressure physically, and the bladder would fill swiftly with no room to store it, so that the pee comes out rapidly, wherever they are, whenever they are feeling that tension.

Osteoarthritis is very probable in 90 percent of all older animals over the age of 12. Much of the breakdown in an animal that is older is bilateral, so they aren't going to look completely lame. With a discerning eye, you will see a little hitch in the giddy-up.

Unless an animal is a complainer (which most cats are not) or there is a lot of licking on a paw to indicate some pain or tissue damage, you might never know. Animals are stoic. They must be. Unless you are the apex predator, you are predator or prey. Dogs and cats in their wildest form are predators until they get old, and then, like the rest of us, they are prey. So, they don't complain."

Humans often jump to the conclusion that inappropriate peeing has behavioral causes. The truth is that much of it is not, and sadly, many animals end up not only in the shelter but euthanized because they are misdiagnosed.

One of the most horrifying reasons for inappropriate peeing in cats is the aftermath of a barbaric practice called declawing. Declawing is, in fact, amputating the top digit. Imagine taking off the top of your finger at the first joint! It's mutilation. The physical stress of being that debilitated would result in a need to express urine. Animals don't blame, this is strictly a stress reaction to a physical compensation.

Urination challenges remain a big challenge for dogs as well. Humans have lots of ways of handling this—belly bands, training, and of course pee pads.

Whether it is a dog or cat, when it comes to "inappropriate" peeing—in my years as an animal communicator—I have found worry to be an underlying emotion that accompanies peeing. With big change, often the household shifts a bit, and the animal may feel displaced or threatened as to their position in their everyday domestic life. There may also be conflict with other animals in the household, which would lead to anxiety and frustration. Marking can be a way of saying "I am not safe." Or for an intact male it could be "Hey, I'm available on Tinder, and you?" If an animal is "excitement-peeing," it is just that. The animal is excited and can't control itself. Usually, they outgrow this, but not overnight. Yet, with all of it, it can be behavioral and/or emotional but it often is accompanied with a physical feeling of pressure in the body that it must come out now.

Second Chakra Emotions and Energetics

The second chakra represents reproduction, creativity, sex, and power, and all one-on-one connection. That connection includes romance, friendship, work relationships, and associations. Second chakra is still waters that run deep. Those deep emotions. So deep they are often overlooked because it is so uncomfortable. Emotions so deep that it could also be delicious to bite in and deal with what comes. Those emotions that could be expanding or contracting. The second chakra is also the deep contract that exists between two beings that are in relationship with one another.

Through the school, Communication with all Life University (CWALU), we always say that there are no good or bad, no positive or negative emotions. All emotion is welcome and necessary for every individual soul and our collective growth. Emotions can be expanding or contracting. Contraction is often where we learn the most in order to expand. Think of inhale, exhale. We can't live in an inhale, and we can't live in an exhale. We need to experience all emotions for balance, harmony, and evolution. The second chakra teaches us this.

In the second chakra, we bury secrets (contraction). Often, these buried secrets here in the second chakra are later revealed in illness, or sexual or hormonal dysfunction. The shadow side—for humans—is codependency, being too emotional, too sensitive, and promiscuous. It is about shame and blame, particularly about sexuality and sexual activity. Yet most of the emotions here, for the most part, are not exactly secret. The primary emotions here are shock, fear, and anger.

Second chakra depth is expressed in pure life force. It is also all about creativity and the birth of a creative endeavor. The physical womb literally expresses breath in the form of new life. The second chakra carries that signature charisma that has taken lifetimes to develop. It is that deep personal triumph, the kind that feels like it is a continuum emerging despite tragic setbacks.

For animals the second chakra also represents sex, power, and one-on-one relationships with their human, and with all others. This includes their one-on-one relationships with other animals in the home, barn, or field, as well as with their medical caretakers, dog walkers, horse trainers, cat groomers, etc. As discussed earlier in this chapter, that "sex and power" in our domestic animals has its limits.

Second chakra for animals invites us humans to understand how fluid feelings and emotions truly are. Animals can go between fixed emotions, meaning contraction or expansion, in two seconds flat because they live in the moment. If they live in a traumatized zone, that is a different story and then trauma is the lens that they look through.

For animals, the core emotions of the second chakra are shock, fear, and anger. Also, these animals tend to be codependent, fixated, have poor boundaries, tend to be too emotional, and too sensitive.

At the dog park we can see the expansive to contracted emotions at work. We watch as all the dogs are super excited and everything is fun until one dog is a little nervous, then they all turn nervous. Tails are waving back and forth, teeth are showing, a little growling, and it becomes a pack-up situation in a minute, and nobody could have predicted it.

A cat can be in a total seeking mode, blissed out, and then, out of nowhere, hear a startling sound. They turn into a hovercraft with a flat tail running to the nearest hiding place and are shaking in fear within a minute.

We can watch passion turn to anger, even violence, and submission become a demand from a hot and heavy stallion in a matter of minutes. We see animals move between these emotions in seconds flat.

If any chakra takes on the mental, emotional, and physical human story, this is the chakra where an animal may get hooked into our crap. What does that look like? Well, a shaman would say there are cords between the human and the animal that would be unhealthy and need to be cut. Because our animals spend so much time trying to please us or worrying about us, for them to see us in these states—angry, fearful, shocked, filled with guilt and shame—they might "attach" to our feelings and become hooked.

Remember, animals are feeling into their pack, herd, pride, flock, colony for survival. If something doesn't feel safe from the leader of the household, well then it really must not be safe. We see this play out in the third chakra more. But the tentacles of codependence and, "Am I safe? Uh oh!!" get installed right into the second chakra.

On the more expanded side of things, the beauty of the second chakra is that animals reflect back to us the amazing, groovy being that we are. They see us as so great, so powerful, so able, so everything. We are the agent of change in their world. They will lift their leg for wound healing because they know we will fix it. They will lay with us because they know we truly "see" them. We are often their world. Or at least the sunshine in it.

When I lived outside of Seattle, you would have thought I ordered the snow specifically for my dog Olivia. I would open the front door to the sight of fresh snow in the morning and she would look at me with sincere gratitude as she flew out of the house to create the first tracks early in the morning as we'd go to feed horses.

The Sheldrick Trust in Kenya is an organization committed to the rehabilitation of orphan elephants. These orphans spend time at the nursery and then, as they become juveniles, the orphan elephants are moved to camps like Ithumba, where they can hang out for the rest of their lives or, they can move into wild herds. It is a beautiful process that occurs through exposure, allowance, and walking through the bush.

There are three "paddocks" at Ithumba and the other "juvenile" camps. One is for the fresh orphans as they create a herd. The middle camp is the herd that is being established, and the third camp is a very established herd that has the opportunity to move into the wild herd. Every morning after their breakfast, the herd goes on a walk through the bush with the trained staff. They often encounter wild elephants and get to know them.

The third grouping of elephants, the more established herd, may veer off with wild herds. Their door is left open at night. Sometimes, a few juveniles will "sneak out" and find the wild herd and hang with them for a few days until they feel like they should go home. And then they sneak out for a few more days with the wild herd until they make that their family.

One of the most profound things about this is, those "orphans" who have been rewilded will come back to the humans at the camp and show off their babies. Or they will come back when they are injured. They even bring injured wild elephants who have no reason to trust humans back to the camp. The wild elephants trust the rewilded elephants and a bond of trust and healing is created.

While we don't want to ever interfere with nature, this is a relationship built out of necessity. And because it is done so carefully, those elephants always know they have a backup. They are also able to show their appreciation by showing up for those touchstone moments.

Nobody Installed the Guilt, Blame, and Shame Button in Animals

We love to think animals feel guilty about the things they do. Maybe in a rare occurrence, they feel guilt. But the truth is, that "guilt" look is simply an energetic reaction to how you're feeling about their behavior. They get how we are feeling before we do!

The joy of going through the garbage far outweighs any punishment for a dog. A cat dangling on the curtains is having so much fun, regardless of how you feel. And wait, you added a water feature, a spray bottle? FUN ALL AROUND. A horse sneaking under the fence for green grass was worth every cuss word they endured. And the entertainment of watching you fix the fence? Worth the price of admission.

Years ago, a friend of mine, Paula, called and said she wanted to set up an animal communication phone consultation for her dog. I said "Paula, you don't need to." "Why not?" she asked. I said, "Because I already know what is going on." Not that I'm that psychic," mind you—but as an Animal Communicator I've seen this a million times. I continued, "You're calling me because your dog is depressed." She agreed. "She came to you depressed and fearful, and you are depressed at times, so the two of you are in the funhouse mirrors right now. She commiserates when you're depressed. When you're not depressed, you spend the rest of the time feeling sorry for her past." I told her to call me in a few days if she still wanted a session.

I explained to my friend that at that point, that dog was lucky. In fact, it had been lucky for all the years they were together. It no longer had the sad circumstances it had before and certainly, over the years, she has expressed her grief and in fact, she has a great life. The dog had a kid and a cat to look after, my friend loves her—it doesn't get any better.

When I saw Paula weeks later, I asked about the dog. She said the switch was overnight, once she had acknowledged that this was a great life. Now, the dog could enjoy life. Not everything is that quick, but really it could be. This is not to say that we need to be in denial, it's the opposite. By staying in the past feelings, we are denying them the present.

When we default into certain second chakra feelings like guilt and worry, we allow the animal to "get away" with certain behaviors that are not serving the harmony of the household. Ultimately, some of these behaviors create dangerous situations. I have seen this over the years around animals that have been rescued from tragic beginnings, or were sick early on.

If we continue to feel sorry for someone, it's like painting on a sticky coat of suffocating sympathy. We are not allowing them to be all that they can be. We are not seeing them as able, not giving them full agency. We are maybe not even fulfilling our contract to hold each other up.

When we hang on to this rescuer/hero/victim story, we don't see who they are. Therefore, we can't even see who they could become. I have seen this time and time again. It is truly the lion's share of an animal communicator's job, helping people get present, seeing the animal's essence of who they truly are, and allowing the animal to blossom.

And unlike humans, animals don't blame. They may get triggered by a guy with a hat because something happened with a guy with a hat. But they aren't saying "Yeah, that asshole kept me in a crate twelve hours a day." They loved that guy even if things weren't stellar. As an onlooker, we may think those things about the guy.

I recently had a student, Natalie, who shared with the class that her dog let her know every single day that he was missing out on the action from the streets and that he preferred his freedom. But rather than being a free-range dog in the small town he lived in, he slept safely under Natalie's desk in her environmental law firm. She feels better about his safety, but he loved his roaming days. She always says her dog's worst day ever was when she "rescued" him from the streets of Mexico.

Years ago, I was teaching animal communication at Stephens College. Aside from being my *alma mater*, it is a wonderful place for animal lovers. I was able to ride through college because they have an awesome equestrian department. Stephens College became one of the first pet-friendly schools by allowing animals in the dorms. And they have a foster program for those who didn't bring their family animal to school.

I taught a mini class for the foster program. One woman had a shy, terrified little white dog stuffed in her armpit under her jacket. To look at this dog, you would think this nervous little dog couldn't survive in the world. The student had been fostering her for a week and shared that this little dog had come from a hoarding situation, and she had been terrified of everything.

We put the little dog up front and center, in front of the students. I led a meditation before we were to communicate with her. Before the meditation, this dog only exhibited anxiety for the first few minutes. She looked down, appeared sad, and seemed unable to care for herself. After the meditation, she was breathing more calmly. I moved everyone into the animal communication. These were beginners, mind you, but when we shared what we received from the session with the dog, we all heard the same thing. Diva. To look at her after she announced her true self, we watched a pathetic little white dog transform between our very eyes into a movie star. She didn't even want to leave the stage; she had become enamored with the attention.

Second Chakra Behavior, Dynamics, and Relationships

The first three chakras are true harbingers of the safety factor, the fight, flight, freeze, or flee. This part of the body really plays out what could be going on for an animal and their ability to handle stress. The more work we are doing to keep the household calm and neutral—alongside introducing confidence-building activities—the better the lives of our animals can be.

We can look at the behavior of an animal in our care, and we can pick apart the dynamics amongst the members of our household. But in truth, our relationship with and for them is really what much of a shift can hinge upon. At some point, whether they are the soulmate, the heart animal, or just one of the herd that we've adopted, there is a karmic contract that lives here in the second chakra between each individual relationship. Particularly us as the human with the animal.

There's a saying when someone is sitting with someone in hospice or going to euthanize their beloved, that we are "walking them home." Well in the meantime, while we are here, perhaps we are just walking each other around. And how did we get chosen for this? I have to believe that, in the grand scheme of things, we created a floodproof contract that we are just blundering through. Somehow at the etheric water cooler where we came up with this soul-to-soul handshake deal, this game plan emerged where we signed on as the "guardian" and they chose "animal companion." The unwritten law here is that, as guardians, we must step into being the emotional leader on occasion.

When we don't take their behavior so personally, we often can create a neutral lens to witness and observe through. And then, we can really see them and view it from their vantage point. We want to consider the emotional life of the animal, the relationship(s) currently, their history, and any dynamics they are playing out with others in the household.

You can work with the Emotional Freedom Technique (EFT) or tapping on the following behaviors:

- Reactivity
- Fear
- Protection
- Pain
- Outer, over or zero stimulation
- Peeing, marking, and more
- Other unwanted behaviors
- Separation anxiety
- Performance blocks

- Working animals (therapeutic riding centers, guide dogs, etc.)
- Show ring, competition

Horse, dog, cat, and bird all have different ways of expressing their reactivity. You can find more on this in my book *Emotional Freedom Technique for Animals*.

When you are really able to discover the origin of the behavior, as in: What are the true feelings here? Is it abject fear? Are they protecting food? Are they protecting an injury? Are they bored out of their mind? then you can understand them better and you can help set up the safety zone and eliminate the triggers.

Some simple questions which could help enlighten why the reactive or anxiety-ridden behavior is happening:

- How many households has this animal been in?
- How much armor from heartbreak is this animal carrying?
- How many people have come and gone?
- How many animals have come and gone?
- How many animals have taken all the great jobs?

Simple questions for yourself are:

- Do I feel sorry for this animal?
- Am I taking their behavior personally?
- Is there a "job" I could give them that would help them to feel like they have purpose?
- Are there ways I've set up an "off" time, away from the others so that they can relax?
- Are they able to self-soothe?

We will go into this more in the third chakra. For now, these are great questions to ponder as you read through the stories. The more an animal feels safe and gets used to that as the norm, rather than fear or chaos, the healthier—mentally, physically, and emotionally—the animal will become.

Stories

Violet

It was 2003, on March 19th. I know because on the radio on the way to the farm, I heard we were bombing Iraq. I had to work extra hard that day to be neutral. The work paid off. I went out to a farm call to talk to horses at a riding center. The owner of the stables, Candy, had me communicate with her own personal animals at the end of the day. Candy had lovely, well cared-for animals but the last horse she brought me to communicate with was her daughter Ann's horse. The stall was the closest to the house. The horse, Violet, was visibly depressed. Candy had only told me that since her daughter had gone off to college, she had hoped to breed Violet, but Violet had not gone into heat for nearly two years. I got quiet to communicate with Violet.

Violet was a beautiful chestnut quarter horse. She was all muscle but, also, all legs. She was a true specimen of beauty. Yet, she was bereft. Violet shared that Ann left for college two years ago, and that since then there had been a fight of some sort; Ann had left college but would not return home. Violet expressed that both she and Candy could do nothing about it, they were helpless. She said both she and Candy were truly bereft. Violet shared more with me about her essence—who she truly is—and what she loves to do. But it didn't feel like both mom (Candy) nor Violet (horse) had expressed the depths of their individual grief. Nor had they both acknowledged their combined grief and disappointment.

When I shared all of this with Candy, she released quite a few tears as she verbally validated Violet's story. Violet also had tears in the corners of her eyes. Candy filled in the details of Ann's addiction and that nobody had heard from her for a long time. Candy shared that it was almost too hard to look at Violet. Candy didn't want to let her go but as a working riding center, Violet should have some purpose. She thought breeding Violet would give them both a purpose. Violet couldn't be bred because she hadn't gone into heat.

I casually placed my hands over the second chakra, feeling into whether or not there was a sacrum challenge, and also in the hopes of finding some flow in the fluids. I have had a fair amount of training in certain body works and particularly cranial/sacral and I love to place my hands on the second chakra of animals.

So, there I was in this stall with a horse that hadn't gone into heat for nearly two years, a grieving mother over an addictive daughter, and the horse that was equally bereft over her loss as she was carnage in Ann's addiction story; then whoosh! I *mean* whoosh, ocean waves of whoosh. Violet went into heat within minutes of placing my hands there. And when a horse goes into heat, there are a lot of fluids released in the form of urine and blood. Violet hadn't been in heat for two years. A grief veil lifted, and a window of possibilities opened. Violet was officially in heat. She was willing to move forward in her journey of shared loss with Candy.

Stanzi

Stanzi was a cat I met in Los Angeles in the late 1990s. She was a gorgeous, vivacious 18-year old with some conditions, both physical and emotional, that seemed to blend. Stanzi had moved across the country from New York City with her person, Audrey. She had basically gone from being the only cat, to one of two cats, to one of four cats within a very short period of time and then had moved across the country to Los Angeles. Archetypally she had gone from Diva to Matriarch, not a chosen path. She barely accepted the brother she had gained in NYC but the two new brothers that were adopted just prior to the move to Los Angeles was hardly tolerable.

Stanzi had been so close to Audrey. She had been a true "mini-me" to Audrey. Stanzi was a wild-hearted woman, just like Audrey had been. Through the years in NYC, Audrey had experienced passionate love and terrible love loss. Audrey had career ups and career downs. She was ready for a fresh start. Audrey was transitioning from being an actress and musician in New York City and moved to Los Angeles because she had been accepted into a prestigious acupuncture school. Audrey would be calling forth a different side of herself, her very feminine, nurturing, healing side. This is where the relationship between Audrey and Stanzi started to shift. Stanzi liked being a wild woman diva. She didn't feel that she had signed up for the matriarch of these new cats. And her second chakra structure was giving way. Her hips literally gave out, and she was dragging her left hind leg.

While it was easy for Stanzi to tolerate the one brother and ignore the other two cats, it was not easy to ignore a leg that wasn't working. Being the true healer that she is, Audrey realized that it was a matter of a little bodywork . . . gently popping the hips back in to get the hind legs back up again. We did animal communication sessions to create peace between all beings, we did lots of scalar wave energy healing to calm the household but, most importantly, Audrey recognized who Stanzi is in her world.

Every time that Audrey did her bodywork, Stanzi was racing around again and was the—elder—wild woman. But the true beauty of this relationship evolution was, in the old days, Stanzi (not unlike Audrey) was a true hellion, had a lot of pride and would never ask for help, let alone accept it. Now Stanzi was presenting her condition and asking for help, and Audrey would offer the help. In the end, when she got going again, she was racing around. They continued to have a beautiful exchange until Stanzi's last breath.

In the end, Stanzi wasn't so bothered by the other animals in her household. She didn't see this as a threat to her relationship with Audrey. She was "with" Audrey in her own unique way of transitioning out of who they each were in New York City—brazen artist rock stars into quiet healer-nurturer Goddesses. Stanzi's implicit trust in Audrey throughout the shifts of her relationship and their household led to her safety even when Audrey was out, and Stanzi's hind end was dragging. Stanzi trusted Audrey to come home, to literally prop her back up, and be on top of the world again. Stanzi held her own with the other cats so that her position of power didn't change even though her physical prowess was diminished. This is a beautiful second chakra phenomenon.

"Honor each other" is what Caroline Myss calls this chakra. I'm game. How about you?

THE THIRD CHAKRA— AWARENESS

"Third chakra energy, the energy of the Personal Power chakra, becomes the dominant vibration in our development during puberty. It assists us further in the process of individuation, of forming a 'self,' ego, and personality separate from our inherited identity. This energy center also contains most issues related to the development of personal power and self-esteem."

—Caroline Myss, Ph.D., *Anatomy of the Spirit: The Seven Stages of Power and Healing*

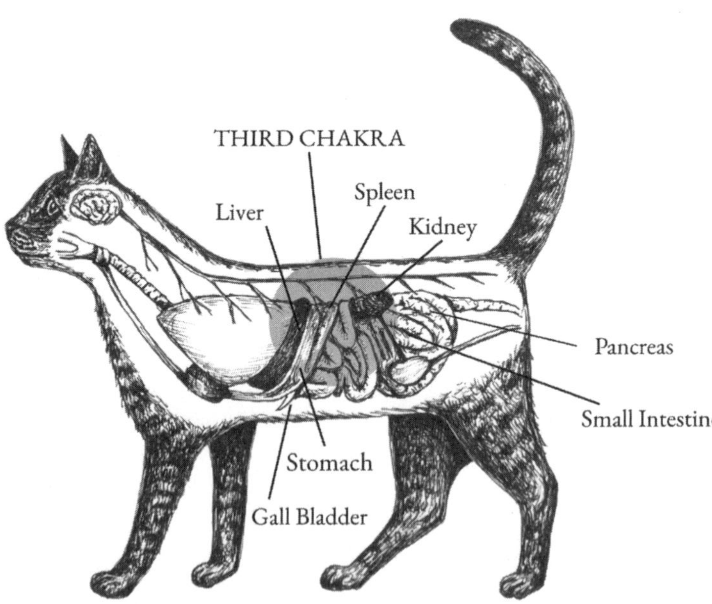

Fig. 4: The third chakra (solar plexus chakra)

Westminster Woofs—Best in Show!

After nearly 150 years, the Westminster Kennel Club Dog Show continues as a tradition at Madison Square Gardens in New York City. The 2022 show was a lively gathering as Westminster dog show goes, meaning the passion was palpable. Even Covid couldn't stop the seats from being full. It was standing room only with a lively crowd that clapped and whistled for each of the contenders of the Best in Show. Seven dogs compete for this final title. The seven dogs were the Best in Show of their category: the terrier group, toy group, working group, sporting group, hound group, non-sporting group, and herding group.

Would judging this be subjective? Normally, I would say yes. They all look fabulous and have beautiful carriage, meaning their gaits delivered perfection for their physical form and athleticism. Each dog certainly checked all the boxes in their breed standard. They had all won so many titles to get to this show and then the ultimate, they were chosen in their category to get to this class: Best in Show. The judge would touch the dog and test the quality, again, seemingly subjective. Yet, this time, something happened. I actually saw it with my own untrained, mutt-loving dog eyes.

The first in, River, the winner of the herding dog category, was a beautiful German shepherd. In comes the winner of the working group, running in sync with his handler. And then, in comes the winner of the hound group, Bloodhound, Trumpet, catching a little air with each bouncy step. And it's done. No matter how perfectly pleasing the Setter is or the stride of the Terrier or how fluffy the Samoyed is, or how joyful the non-sporting French Bulldog (who is so famous) or how the Maltese moves without shaking her locks, nobody could out do "something" in Trumpet's beingness.

With the anticipation and intensity of the selection process you have to wonder, what was it? What is it? The judge says, "Thank our dogs for the comfort, joy and love they give us," and then announces the reserve, and finally Best in Show: Trumpet. Then the camera shows Trumpet running in slow motion and those jowls and long floppy ears flow from side to side, taking up the entire screen.

What exactly was the "it" factor? Was it his looks? Was it that there was a hint in his aura of a giant goofball? Was it his sparkling personality? The jowls? The ear length?

Ultimately, why would I open a third chakra animal chapter with a competition? The truth is, I have several reasons. The first and foremost is that competition, like bloodwork, is a way in which humans measure things about animals. Granted, it is our measurement, but many, or enough of them, certainly go along with it.

Secondly, they compete on their own, often just for fun. Having had thoroughbreds most of my life, if you have two males in a pasture, someone is going to start a race and someone is going to win. And it is usually the same dude that started the race.

Thirdly, through healthy competition or boundary testing, they create status, hierarchy or, at the very least, they test to make sure those boundaries are solid.

Boundaries are a very important part of the third chakra because if someone isn't seen, heard, acknowledged, or able to take care of themselves within the herd, pack, pride, or our dog and pony show homes, they may end up suffering for it later, physically.

Third Chakra Symbolism

When does a personality start? How is it shaped? Is it all soul? Is the soul the collective experience that then informs the environment? Or does the environment inform the soul? Does the soul come in and say, "I need this experience; therefore, I will be this personality and just work through my stuff?" What determines who we are? Is it nurture or nature?

In the human world, the third chakra represents confidence, self-esteem, and personal power. It is the center of identity, the seat of the ego, and strength. It also holds our anger. It is the blueprint for self-acceptance, peace, and that true sense of self.

And the third chakra is literally the filter, how we take in, digest the world. It is our gut instinct. It is that gnawing tummy ache, the butterflies when "something just aint right."

For animals, the third chakra is all of those things too. The filter, the gut, the instinct moving from the gut into action. The first and second chakra are so primary in fight or flight, but the third chakra really is that bridge between instinct, personality, and interfacing with the rest of the world. The third chakra starts to feel the world. The third chakra for animals is awareness.

Some scientists argue that animals don't have a personality or a sense of self. Obviously, nobody reading this would be of that school of thought. But the third chakra, the stomach, is the key to the personality, even in the wild.

They say that personality, or a sense of self, is defined by having a sense of future outcomes. Animals literally have a sense of their future based on their past because of their gut. If an animal out in the wild has ever experienced a storm, 12 to 15 hours before the storm hits, they sense the barometric pressure change in their gut.

They start moving to higher ground. They start moving to places of protection among trees, in canyons, etc. They have had an experience in the past that tells them that they don't want to be in the open, they will be too vulnerable. Therefore, based on their past, they are shaping their future. That awareness starts in the gut and creates the instinct to protect themselves.

It also starts to define their emotions and metabolism. But more on that later.

Do Animals Have an Awareness?

Awareness in the wild and at home is experienced, even when nobody is looking! Awareness comes in all forms.

- Awareness in nature
- Awareness in the home
- Awareness in the show ring
- Awareness if you are the runt
- Awareness if you are part of family—even if you are part of a boarding situation
- Awareness of affection and the need to receive and express it—even if your body is too big to fit in the lap anymore
- Awareness of the way others treat you
- Awareness of boundaries

Ironically, even though this is the last of the 3 chakras that are more instinctual or even carry the primitive sense of fight, flight, fright or freeze, this chakra has a placeholder in the map of the body as the first step in awareness. And in part because of their gut and ability to respond.

Awareness, sentience, and consciousness are all connected. Consciousness would imply an awareness of all that is going on in and around a being. The internal sensations and emotions as well as aware spatially.

Do animals have a Spiritual awareness? Spiritual awareness is said to be the soul's intelligence. I think that is as individual as the being is. Some may have more; some may have less. If we were to apply the human spirituality, this would suggest that this would be part of the evolution of each particular soul.

I spent much of my education in a private Catholic girl's school called Forest Ridge. It was run by the nuns of the Sacred Heart. I had some very jagged questions in religion class, in particular, about two very pressing interchangeable things. This is at age six. Mind you, these two questions continued on throughout my stay at this school, and my life:

1. My animals: Sister Pimento, are you absolutely positive our animals don't have souls?
2. I was always concerned for my non-Catholic friends: Would they also be going to heaven?

Is it any wonder that I was kicked out in the ninth grade after spending my life there?

In the last few years, the Pope has assured us that animals have souls. Nobody needed the Pope to assure this because we all know this.

Like humans, some animals may have a personal mission that takes over. Sometimes that mission gives them the profound sense of self and fulfills their sense of purpose.

Awareness brings on the question of ego. Could an animal have ego? Some argue: Animals live in the moment; therefore, an ego is out of the question. But even if they live seemingly moment, to moment, they have recognition of experiences. If I put my dogs in the car and drive toward the beach, my dogs are amped up and ready to go shred the sand up and body surf the waves, 20 twenty minutes before I get to the parking lot.

Some animals are aware that you are not aware! People love to think that their animal is protecting them when their animal is reactive. The truth is that the animal is protecting him/herself because they are very aware of the fact that their human is distracted, or not leadership material.

If the boundaries aren't put into place, an animal can run the house and it can appear to be ego-driven or arrogant when it is truly a profound sense of self without boundaries. All cultures, no matter what species, have some sort of groundwork laid out about the hierarchy of who is what and in what capacity. Yet, we anthropomorphize situations like when the cat bullies everyone. It isn't his ego; it is his bigger-than-life sense of self without anyone else laying down the law.

That profound sense of self can also work in the way of being very Zen and calming everyone down. The cat who seems to philosophize while sitting in the window. The horse who calms the whole herd down. The dog that has a way of stopping the fight between other dogs. These are all things we would assign to the personality, the persona, the essence of that animal. All of those qualities live largely in the third chakra.

The Chakra Systems of Animals and Humans

The chakra system of a human correlates with that of an animal covering the same areas and organs within the body. Below you'll find the names and locations of the seven chakras discussed in this book:

- First Chakra – Muladhara: "Root" – base of the spine
- Second Chakra – Svadhishthana: "Where the self is established" – sacral/under the belly button
- Third Chakra – Manipura: "Jewel City" – solar plexus
- Fourth Chakra – Anahat: "Unstruck" – heart center
- Fifth Chakra – Vishuddha: "Purest" – throat center
- Sixth Chakra – Ajna: "Command" – brow/third eye
- Seventh Chakra – Sahasrara: "Thousand-Petaled" – crown

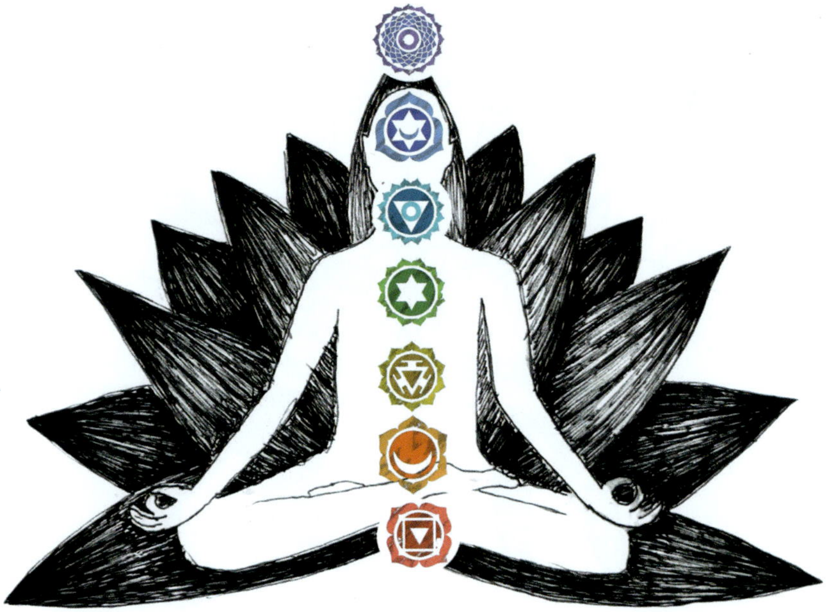

The 7 Chakras of a Human

The images below provide an overview of which body areas are covered by which chakra in various animals.

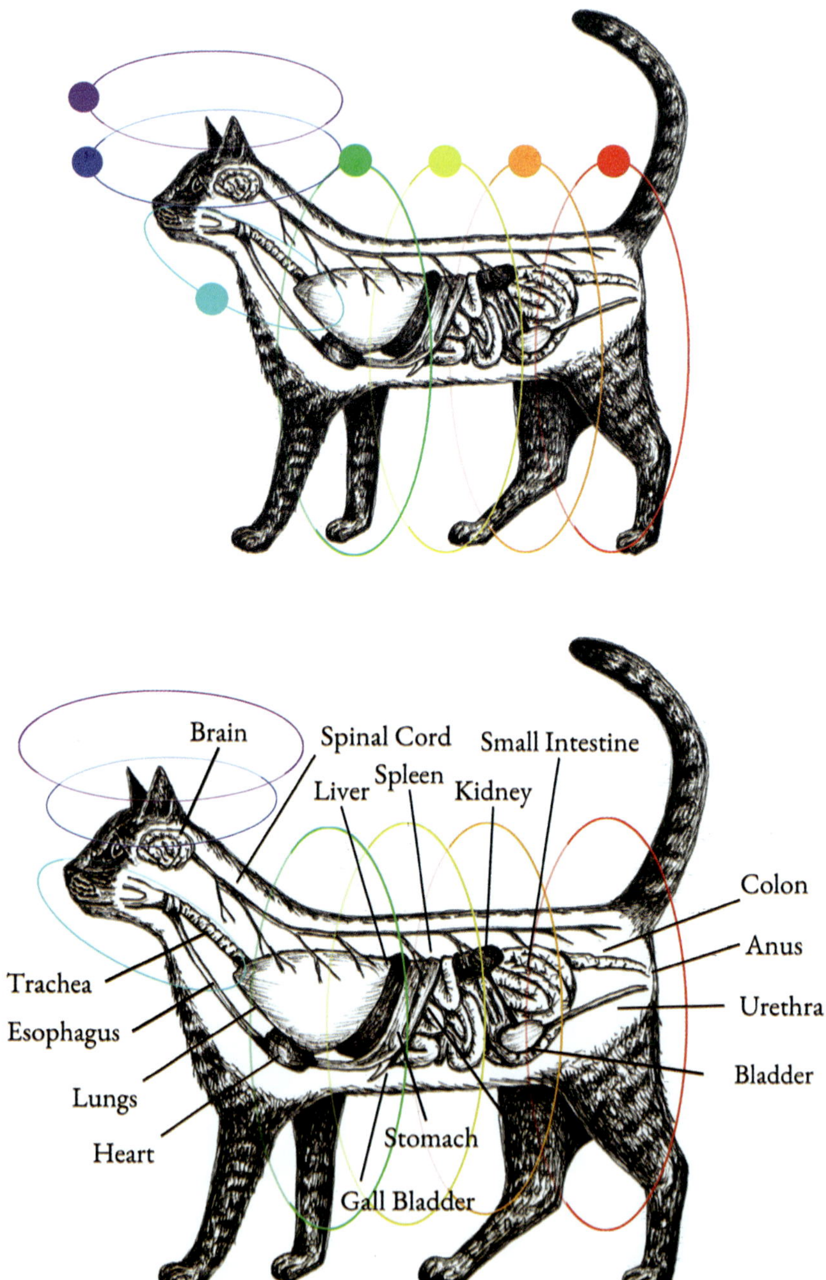

The 7 Chakras of a Cat

The 7 Chakras of a Horse

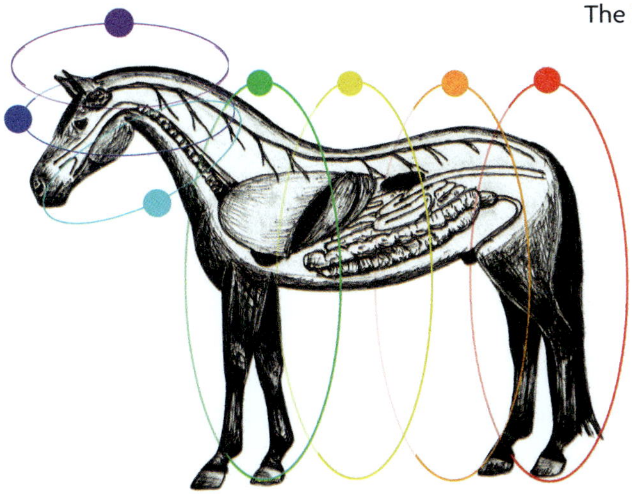

The 7 Chakras of a Chicken

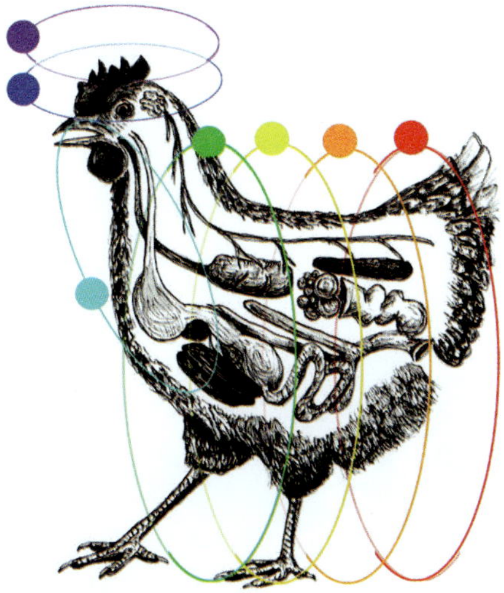

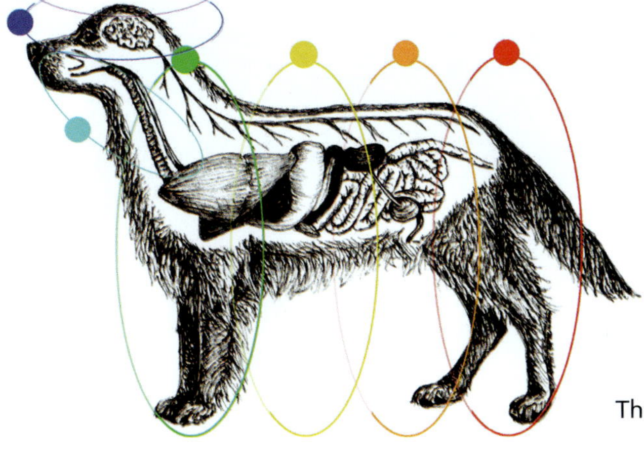

The 7 Chakras of a Dog

With consent from the animal, it is always lovely to connect up with the physical body by placing one hand over the second chakra (hips) and the other hand over the heart chakra (base of the neck). As you place your hands here, just breathe for a moment. Allow your breath to follow along with the inhales and exhales of the animal, so you sync up with them.

If you can't touch the animal or you are working remotely, imagine you are connecting up the second and fourth chakras with your hands in the same way but without touching. It's as if your hands are feeling into the whole system, the chakras, the meridians, the nervous system, and more.

Below you see the chakra points directly on the body.

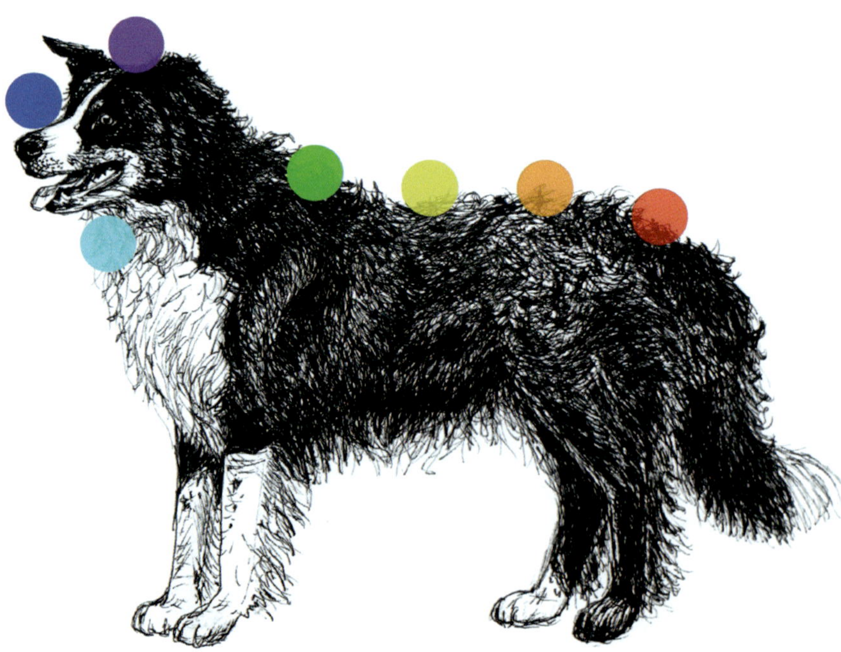

The Chakra Points on the Animal Body

In my school, Communication with all Life University (CWALU), we teach animal communication by discovering who they are through telepathy. Telepathy is the transference of pictures, words, and feelings. We all do it all the time! While it sounds complex, it is deceptively simple. After a little meditation, we ask the animal who they are by way of their "essence." The essence is who they are at their core, their spirit, how their heart/soul expresses themselves. As beings, their purpose, their trajectory, their wounding, their healing, their throughline through lifetimes is recognized, and can transform here in the third chakra. We also find out their favorite things to always be able to provide joy and let their beingness be fully realized.

Third Chakra Species-Specific/Wild and Domestic

The third chakra interacts daily like a homing device. Our gut tells us, "This is bad, this is bad, step away. No touching. Move away." Or, "Awwwww, this is nice. We can stay here a minute. This feels good. This is so gooooood." This is our gut instinct literally and figuratively. The third chakra is how we absorb and metabolize the world, and therefore how we respond or react to the data. And for animals, there is very little filter involved. Meaning, as humans, we may hold back and not say what we mean. But animals are truth and presence. The gut will inform their reaction to everything whether it is "Uh oh," or "Awwwwww."

That said, they do know how to mask to survive. In a herd, a pack, or a pride, the elder that is weak will be pushed out eventually or they will opt to move themselves out to not burden the group. But in our homes, they can't do that in quite the same way. Our domestic friends can mask and sometimes the other animals recognize that they are weaker and push them out. We humans do not always have the same kind of awareness to recognize when our animals are masking their getting ill or weaker.

The third chakra awareness is both a physical and emotional reality when it comes to fight or flight. It's like an emotional alarm goes off in the gut and a physiological volcano fires off from the adrenals. The lungs expand to run faster, the brain is focused, and they are off to safety. Hopefully.

Animals have a twenty-four-hour weather channel in their guts. Out in the wild, they can feel barometric pressure change hours before the weather changes and find higher ground. Most of us have walled off our guts to such an extent that we aren't even aware we have digestive issues, let alone a weather detector!!

A dog that is affected by thunder and lightning can sometimes feel them approaching 8 to 12 hours before they first strike. We don't notice but then we see our animal is seeking sanctuary in the porcelain bathtub or shoe closet. They are taking control of their future based on their past because their stomach is letting them know.

Our animals can often be a great dating service. Meaning, when you bring someone new home, your animals will often react either favorably or be wary. This is their gut at work. You can thank them later.

The Shadow Side of the Third Chakra

The shadow side of this chakra in its simple form is anxiety, feeling invisible, and lack of self-esteem.

Because the third chakra involves self-esteem, we can see our animals languish or get caught up in unwanted behavior because they have lack of confidence or aren't fully aware of boundaries. We can see a lot of separation anxiety, or anxiety in general, that stems from this chakra.

Many horses have saddle issues in that area. Dogs can have mid-back issues and lose strength in this area as they age. Cats end up with kidney disease.

Here are some emotional/energetic scenarios that could lead to a breakdown in the third chakra:

- Animals that have been rehomed repeatedly.
- Horses that have changed jobs several times.
- Animals that are newly adopted when the grief of the former animal hasn't quite subsided.
- The family dog that has watched the kids it helped raise go off to college.
- Animals that are picked on by other animals.
- Animals that were not treated kindly in human households and are now scarred by insecurities.
- The kick-me sign, the animal with the repeated patterns, owner after owner.
- The kick-me sign, the animal with the repeated patterns of getting beat up by other animals.
- The stoic animal that won't let on it is in greater pain than it lets on.

This list represents just a few of the common issues that might drive a breakdown in this area.

Things that could quickly support an animal who experiences mental, emotional, or physical challenges in this area include:

- Recognizing and appreciating whatever job the animal in your household is doing.

- Reassigning jobs when big changes are made in a household to help the animal retain a sense of security.
- Letting new animals know that they are loved.
- Allowing moments for the animal at the bottom of the pecking order to just breathe and be themselves.
- Finding activities that help the animal gain a strong sense of self and its relationship with you.
- Allowing the animal to express itself through play and other joyful activity.
- Playing with archetypes, assigning a new purpose.
- Training.
- Boundaries.
- Exercise, play, laughing, good food, and clean water to support the animal's health.

Note about this chapter: It will appear repetitive when it comes to emotional, energetic, and physical. This is the one chakra that integrates everything and can never be explained enough!

Third Chakra Organs, Structure, Body Parts, and Meridians

Organs

The third chakra sits at the solar plexus and is like the sun shining out. The color is yellow. It governs our stomach, liver, gall bladder, kidney, pancreas, spleen, adrenals, digestion, filtering organs, and glands. The small intestine lives here which is broken into the duodenum, jejunum, ileum, cecum, and part of the colon. The third chakra is all about the digestion and absorbing nutrients.

Well-known holistic physician Dr. Andrew Weill considers the stomach "the second brain."

- Physiological systems at work here: digestive (digest and assimilate), metabolic (utilize energy from food and water), and renal system (excretion of water, regulate fluid).
- Endocrine systems at work here: adrenals and pancreas (pancreas is seen as both an organ and a gland).
- Nerve plexus: Celiac plexus, sits behind the pancreas and speaks to the brain, spinal cord, digestive organs, Peripheral Nervous System (PNS).
- Spine: Lumbar (low back) L1–L5, the largest of the entire spine.

Meridians and Traditional Chinese Medicine

Governing Vessel (GV), Conception Vessel (CV), Stomach (ST), Spleen/pancreas (SP), Kidney (KI), Gallbladder (GB), Liver (LV). Both the Spleen and Liver meridians end in the third chakra area.

Horses do not have a gallbladder, though they still have a gallbladder meridian.

In Traditional Chinese Medicine, the liver is associated with anger, the gallbladder with frustration, the kidneys with fear, the spleen with worry, and the stomach with pensiveness.

- The liver (yin) meridian meets the gallbladder meridian on the foot, travels up the inside of the hind legs and around the belly (on either side), and ends on the lower rib cage.

Putting It All Together: Digestion

This chakra is responsible for digestion in all species. And that means not only the physical digestion, but also our mental and emotional. This is home of the gut instinct. It is about absorbing food, information, and even others' emotions. It is a giant distribution center, as food enters the system and is broken up and sent in all directions to process to aid in energy and growth. If the system is balanced well with nutrition, minerals, vitamins, and hydration, the endocrine system runs more smoothly. And if all of that is running smoothly, there is more mental clarity and emotional stability.

- The stomach is in constant motion to balance the pH (potential of hydrogen), which is a dance between acidity and alkalinity. Balancing food, exercise, mental stimulation, and emotional life is the key to good health. The stomach has so many nerve endings, that it is considered the second brain. Those nerve endings are the communication system between the intestine (including the bacteria), the brain, and the immune system.
- "I" diseases in the gut start here because of too much acidity.
- Animals are in touch with their instincts in a way that humans have lost track of. The main vehicle for their instinctual messages is the stomach. A perfect example is the animal who knows well in advance a storm is coming; it feels the barometric pressure change in its stomach.
- More and more the foods that we are feeding to animals are overly processed. The soil no longer holds the same minerals it once did. All of this contributes to the dulling of the nerve endings and inhibiting the animals' natural instincts. These over-processed and highly chemical-laced foods also constrain the production of

serotonin, which regulates mood, and this can contribute to metabolic disorders. Again, the health and behavior of an animal is intertwined, and the stomach is the center of that.

- Whether it is poor food quality or high emotions, when acidity rises above the alkalinity and isn't balanced, we can see a lot of challenges in health and behavior. Imagine acidity to have a "hot" quality. This is the sensation of a nervous tummy, something an anxious animal would experience. This heat could lead to acid reflux, and it is something that you can literally smell.
- An acidic tummy also leads to all the "I" (inflammation) conditions. Arthritis, colitis, and the list goes on. This acidic tummy is also the underlying situation for leaky gut syndrome, ulcers, IBD, IBS, digestive disorders, autoimmune disorders, and more.
- The third chakra is home to hypoglycemia, insulin resistance, metabolic disorders, and diabetes—losing the "sweetness of life."
- Adrenal fatigue is part of the third chakra. Imagine an animal in constant fight or flight or suffering from anxiety. The adrenals are turned on high like a fire hose.
- Anxiety and nervous tummy can change the neurotransmitter serotonin and alter mood.
- There are amazing resources out there to perfect the animal diet. There has never been a better time to become educated. And it is important to do because great health is more sustainable for the longevity of our animal companions, but it also uses fewer resources. While there may be more of an expense with the food, there is often less of an expense in veterinary care.
- Food and nutrition are some of the most important tools we have to support animal health. Many animals are afflicted by terrible human diseases that can be traced to digestion. Household animal

companions and horses have food allergies, insulin resistance, ulcers, liver disease, and kidney disease, to name a few. We have replicated nearly every possible human disease in our animals because of poor food choices that we are making for them.

- Ulcers, particularly in horses. Worth mentioning again and again.

In my book *Energy Healing for Animals*, I share good lifestyle practices in terms of feeding, and questions to ask yourself about how you want to feed your animals. If you are new to the idea that you may need to change their diet, it is a good resource. And, in the book I bring up "how" we feed our animals.

Cats and dogs are both predators and prey. But when it comes to eating, they are predatory. They would have hunted. All that activity sets the stage for the digestive juices to do their best job. When we make lifestyle choices of leaving food down for them, it is convenient for us but not good for their system.

Horses on the other hand need to be digesting nearly 20 hours out of the 24 hours. They move and graze all day. They used to get the minerals they needed from the soil. In fact, the soil itself worked as a gut cleaner each time a bit of dirt moved through their system with the grasses.

When we truly consider our animals, we have to look beyond our convenience and find a way to meet them where they are. If you don't feel you can prepare raw food for your animal friend, could you feed prepared raw food? Could you investigate the second-best option, cooking for your animal? There are plenty of recipe books available. Finally on my list is food out of a bag or can. And if you must, could you consider adding raw and/or real foods to top-dress this?

Lifestyle plays a key role in the third chakra's health. Self-esteem goes hand in hand with our understanding of the third chakra. Activity, fun, play, good sniffing walks, training, learning something new, allowing our animals to seek and discover things are all part of helping their self-esteem rise. When they are in "rest and digest" and content, they can't be anxious. Therefore, finding this balance is key to their mental, emotional, and physical health.

Third Chakra Emotions and Energetics

In the human world, the third chakra is known for self-esteem and self-worth and the color is yellow. Imagine the tummy is just a little bright sunshine. For animals it is the same thing, but it isn't the beacon the human chakra is, it shines out a little differently.

Emotionally, the third chakra governs self-esteem, gut instincts, gut reactions, and emotional digestion. This area tells animals whether they can trust something or not. The third chakra is like a lens that determines how animals feel and see the world. The world reflects back to them through this chakra as to how they are seen in the world.

This is the center of awareness, exchange, courage, get-up-and-go, and will. It is a true processing center, whether it works on dispensation of nutrients while digesting food, or navigating emotions and all things energy.

In Traditional Chinese Medicine, the liver is associated with anger, the gallbladder is associated with frustration, the kidneys are associated with fear, the spleen is associated with worry, and the stomach with pensiveness.

This location physically is where they read us. This is where they know what is going on with us. Gut to gut. Often this is where we hook into them as well. Meaning, when we are in a relationship battle of wills, much like we can do with a spouse or a child, we are hooked in third chakra to third chakra. This is also the area where we can play ping pong with anxiety. First it is the dog with the nervous tummy, and then it is the person. Or was it the person to begin with? It doesn't matter, it goes back and forth here like a bad bio feedback infinity loop. Until one day the person gets training or goes to therapy and says, "Hey, I want off this roller coaster." And that is when the human steps into what I call emotional leadership.

They hook into our third chakra when we aren't feeling so great. When we lack confidence, they can be very sweet and lick our tears, build us up, give us a look of love. All the while, they are plotting the takeover. Not because of any other reason than they need confident emotional leadership.

If I had a dime for every time someone said to me, "Oh my dog is just protecting me when he gets reactive," I'd be very rich. Then the look on the person's face when the lightbulb turns on after I say to them, "No, your dog is protecting themselves because they don't see you as a strong leader and they don't believe they are safe."

As much as we see the "safety-first" in the first chakra, this is the "companion safety-first" chakra regarding the relationship between animal and human. Animals must feel emotionally safe. When they don't feel safe, they will create their own status, boundaries, and hierarchies. In a pack, pride, flock, herd or murder of crows, there are rules, status, boundaries, birth order, strengths to consider, jobs, and hierarchies. And if there is a weak link, for the purpose of survival, someone will take over.

Anxiety is the one thing that could be considered physiological and emotional. We can see it in their digestion. We can see it in their behavior. And we want to treat both, the gut physically, as well as creating confidence-building activities.

The third chakra is where separation anxiety lives. Dogs can become destructive, howl, pace, bark, urinate, poop, you name it. Cats get destructive. Horses panic. If they are herd-bound, they will neigh and run in circles with their head high in the air. When they experience fear, they often poop loose stools.

Some of the things that enhance their lifestyle and create confidence and healthy self-esteem:

- Nutrition—enough can't be said about a healthy balanced diet for all life!
- Lifestyle—having a happy lifestyle can include activities that the animal companion loves to do as well as having them as companions on activities you love to do. Some dogs like to go along for the ride, so to speak, and that can be a great adventure!
- Exercise—like humans, exercise plays a key role in mental and emotional health.
- Seeking—finding ways for our animals to be able to seek, whether it is sniffing out in the yard, or going on an exploration through the trails. Animals need to have their curiosity piqued. If they are homebodies, hide the treats!
- Training—this is one of the most important things you can do to help an animal be able to have a common language with you. It is not only confidence-building but can have a safety factor to it. If your animals aren't trained and someone had to evacuate your house, what would happen?
- Management—many people are in a situation in which they must manage animals through crate and rotate or keep them in other

rooms because there has been a bloody dispute. This is not the end of the world, rather a safety measure. As long as all of the parties get a little "me" time with their person or other animals, sometimes this is the best way to keep animals safe and in their confidence.

- Animal Communication—I can't even tell you how many times animals have been adopted in shelters after an animal communication session because their essence has been revealed. Everyone heals when they feel acknowledged, their story has been told, and they are seen for who they are. This is the gift of animal communication.
- Energy Healing—this is a very important way of helping an animal get out of rage or shut down to be able to be in their body and be who they are.
- Relationships—animals like and need each other. Humans are okay but they need to be with the same species. Sometimes even the same breed. When my border collie sees other working dogs, she goes crazy in a great way.
- Role models—sometimes your more feral animals need to see it through another animal. A feral cat may settle in faster with another cat. Mustangs need to watch other mustangs who are domesticated. I had a feral dog who learned everything from my other dog.
- Self-soothe—whether it is chewing or licking, find a proactive way to turn an "anxiety" release into a simple self-soothe activity.
- Time out—everyone needs space. Honoring our animals in this way can be very healthy. Wolves and coyotes have a den, lions sleep in a pile—A LOT, and horses take turns napping while out in the wild. Everyone has a time out where there is no pressure

from the other. Unfortunately, we micromanage their lives, not realizing they need to go nap in the other room. Going away for a while is good for them.

Ultimately, we want to support their ability to shine brightly in the world and be confident whether you are home or not. I always say if something happened to me, my animals would be really sad, but they could still thrive. That is my wish for them every day.

Stories

When it comes to the third chakra and behavior, relationships, and dynamics, we can easily point to patterns, belief systems, how thoughts contribute to behavior or self-esteem. Training is one of the many things that helps with confidence in this chakra.

A weakened third chakra is also home to what I refer to as the "energetic kick-me sign." What I mean by that is these animals appear to have a "kick-me" sign on their back that others jump on the band wagon to take them down.

Romeo, Daisy, and Freya

In my Advanced Animal Communication, Behavior, Relationships, and Dynamics class a student, Maria, presented a situation. She shared that she had a younger cat, Romeo, who would beat up the two girl cats, Daisy, and Freya. Daisy and Freya were pretty badass, but when Romeo was around, they were like the epitome of the shrinking violet. I asked Maria if this had happened before with another cat, and she said "Yes!" There had been another cat before, Jack, who beat the girls up daily.

When situations go unnoticed, not managed, or unhealed, the pattern continues and deepens, no matter where the animals go. This is not to blame in any way, sometimes we don't notice the subtleties of the relationships of our animals. Particularly, if we have a few animals, like I do!

Back to the two cats. While this was a pattern our student Maria had now with two bully boys, and two shrinking violets, the bullying likely happened for each of these cats with a perpetrator even before Maria adopted them. This is where animal communication, energy healing, a little training or management is golden, enlightens the guardian to the situation and can offer guidance to shift it.

The Pattern

It seems that the energetic signature of a behavioral pattern that involves self-esteem starts here in the third chakra. It is like a bad bio-feedback loop in the form of an infinity sign going back and forth from each side. Who knows where it begins or ends. Does the animal have low self-esteem and that is why it continues to get picked on, or is the animal picked on once and the low self-esteem develops? That is the question.

Recurring patterns is one of the many reasons that I created the Shelter Initiative, using animal communication and EFT (Emotional Freedom Technique) Tapping to help the animals in the shelter to heal at a core level and create sustainable adoption. By breaking up the patterns, hopefully, animals can land in their next home as a forever home.

Pegasus

Pegasus is the perfect name for that white Arabian horse who looks as though he could sprout wings and run with the wind. He has perfect confirmation, a perfect disposition except for that little defeated look in his eye. Saffyre Sanctuary is a rescue known for being a sanctuary for many older or injured horses who cannot be adopted, but it is also a rescue for elders who can still be placed.

The founder, Esta, came over one day and happened to show me pictures of this beautiful fellow and asked if I knew anyone who was interested in him. I said, "I am."

At the time, I had a small herd of three horses. One of them, Gabrielle—who has been the subject of many stories in previous books—was 36 years old. She was my companion for over 33 years. She was always in and out of "hospice" at this point, having degenerative challenges with her knees and other complications. With only one good leg, she was still fiery.

I thought Pegasus might make a nice equine companion for Gabrielle. She was flanked, literally, by my other horse Anya. Anya would never leave Gabrielle's side unless she was working with me, or Gabrielle was with me. I thought Pegasus would also be a good companion for Anya when the day came that Gabrielle would leave for the Rainbow Bridge.

According to the story, Saffyre was about to take him in because, his person, a man, had died a couple of years ago. The man's widow also had the companion horse. Since her husband's death, the widow was moving the horses from place to place. In part because, no matter what happened, Pegasus was getting beat up by the other horses.

One look at Pegasus and I sensed what was going on. He had what I call the "energetic kick-me sign" pasted right there in his third chakra. If the other horses even looked at him, they could smell his low place in the herd ladder. They could sense his low self-esteem. Yet, humans fell in love with him.

And when he came here, it was no different. My male horse, Drakkar, bit him and drove him away from his girls for a couple of months. That part was no surprise. Drakkar thinks he's the big man on campus. Where would I find all the bite marks? Right there, mid-back, third chakra.

Through time, acceptance, and a lot of EFT (Emotional Freedom Technique) Tapping, I now have a very happy herd. Gabrielle has since crossed over. A new friend, Felina, has joined the herd. Again, there was some excitement and bared teeth from Drakkar. Even some ear pinning by Anya, but nothing like the first few days here, certainly nothing like the sad stories Esta had shared with me and certainly, the sad feeling Pegasus had was shed with the spring coat. He has confidence, he is independent, and part of the herd.

Pegasus is lucky, and so are we! Being aware of these power centers and their vulnerability can have a profound impact on healing. Challenges for some animals become embedded into their systems and are not easy to overcome if not attended to.

Calypso

A woman named Barbara had me out to a barn to meet a horse named Calypso. I met the very fine tall thoroughbred who at one time had raced at the track. The horse was now in a dressage program after being with several people and having had a prior career of three-day eventing (dressage, show jumping, and cross-country jumping). Barbara was convinced that Calypso had been abused.

I connected with him telepathically, writing down everything I got from him, as I do in a session. Some of it makes sense and some of it appears to be random images. I kept getting one image of a trailer. After my initial contact with the animal, I wait for a moment to see if there is anything else the animal wants to communicate, if there is any other information that is going to be downloaded to me for the sake of healing, or if there is a way in which I need to diplomatically convey information to the human.

His way of communicating was pretty straightforward and, as convinced as she was of the abuse, I really didn't sense that. Additionally, he was very unsure of himself in certain areas and the saddle seemed to be an issue. You could also see physically that he was always sizing you up and that the whites of his eyes were quick to flash if he didn't like what you were doing.

I then explained that I had seen a trailer, asked if there had been a trailer accident, and she said not to her knowledge. I then asked Calypso why the trailer kept flashing before me and I got a sense of him hitting his head going in, his hind legs slipping out from under him, sliding under the trailer and the front half of his body was still upright and struggling to get out from underneath the trailer. The more he struggled, the more trapped his hind end got. In the struggle, the area that was completely twisted was the third chakra.

It made sense to Barbara as I could show her the line of where the sciatic nerve was a little tweaked, and poked on the horse's back where the area was that he was twisted. That minor poke nearly sent him to the ground.

All that was great, but Barbara wanted to know more about the abuse. "Well, I didn't necessarily see abuse," I said. Then she said, "I didn't want to say anything, but you know the last person that had him. You've actually talked to him before."

I thought his energy and this trailer story was familiar. Barbara even said you know his old trainer, and she mentioned a friend of mine.

On the drive home I called the trainer and chatted with her. I asked her whether she remembered a super tall horse named Calypso? She said that she did and that I had talked to him. I usually have a good memory, but I have talked to a lot of animals. She described the last owner.

I told the trainer how Barbara was absolutely convinced the last owner had abused him. The trainer told me that the last owner was convinced that the owner before her must have abused the horse. I asked the trainer if she remembered the saddle area being really tender and she said, "Oh yeah, it was very much a tender spot. That's why people were afraid of him because he would buck when he was uncomfortable. You told us about a trailer accident where he got his spine stuck and twisted by being stuck under the trailer. The owner then confirmed that it happened."

So, there it was, again. The trailer accident that this horse was telling me about before, the horse still wanted me to make sure I told Barbara about it.

I share this particular story as an illustration because, the kick-me sign can come in the form of an accident, an attack, an individual not standing up for themselves.

What if it really was an accident in a trailer that has injured that third chakra? What if it really is such deep grief that it has created anxiety? Or ulcers? What if the animal isn't protecting you, but him/herself?

Calypso was sold to one more owner and was eventually euthanized. He had a giant scary buck that not only injured people, but it also terrified them to their core. If someone would have acknowledged his terror from the accident, recognized the soft tissue damage, gotten chiropractic help right away and worked with other energy modalities to take the trauma out of his muscle memory, Calypso wouldn't be a big horse with a kick-me sign on his back. Because in truth, he saw himself as a kind mouse.

Many animals have this "kick-me" sign. We see them at the dog park, they are the first to get attacked. We see them in the home, they are the first animal to get picked on and are in hiding. And we see them in the shelter, they try to go invisible.

The Human Kick-Me Sign

A woman, Iris called because her cat, Chloe was attacking her. Iris had a three-month old baby, so this was concerning. Iris loved Chloe, yet she was concerned for her baby. Chloe had been a feral cat that she rescued and brought into the home. Prior to her human baby, Chloe was the baby. Since the baby was born, Chloe started attacking her.

In the animal communication session, Chloe let me know that she loved Iris. Iris protested immediately, "Why does she attack me?"

I shared that Chloe felt as though Iris expected Chloe to attack her. In many ways, Chloe felt challenged at times. And that challenge was charged. Chloe soon became over-stimulated with touching (as many feral and non-feral cats do). And that Iris was no longer sensitive as to how long the touch could go on.

Suddenly my own intuition kicked in and I asked Iris: "Were you attacked as a kid by a cat?" Iris said yes.

I told her that on some level there were old tapes that were playing in the back of her mind and that Chloe was responding to that "expectation." Accidentally, Iris was making an invitation.

Iris got off the call and I couldn't tell whether it struck a chord, or she wasn't buying it. That night, I got an e-mail from her saying, "You are right, I told my husband about the session, and he said that I used to say: 'Eventually the cat will attack me because cats do.'"

Iris worked through her trauma with cats through EFT Tapping.

Thankfully, Iris had the courage to follow through with the work so that she could let go of that, and she has kept a deep relationship with Chloe and the baby is fine. And the baby is now an adult and a cat lover.

Belief Systems

How we feel about someone can have a direct impact on how they feel about themselves. For this reason, I have a "Poor Baby Fund" going in my school, Communication with all Life University. When we have classes, whether they are live in-person, or on Zoom, students "read" or communicate with animals from a picture.

Diane G would often look at the picture of the animal and, after having heard the story of the animal, whether it was the dog had cancer or the cat was in its second home, Diane would look across at the person and unconsciously, automatically say, "Poor Baby." That is, until I started charging her money!

I finally asked, "Diane, do you realize the energy you are projecting onto this animal?"

The definition of sympathy is "Feelings of pity or sorrow for one's misfortune." Is that helpful? Whereas empathy is "The ability to understand and share the feelings of another." Do you see the difference?

Our perception of pity or sorrow for another usually hits right in the gut. If an animal (or human) is down, sympathy ends up having an adverse effect.

When I started charging twenty dollars in "poor baby" money, my students stopped saying it. For those who did, they contributed to a fund for some of the favorite organizations of the school, like the Gentle Barn, Saffyre Sanctuary, the Gibbon Conservation Fund, and more. It has even become funny with some of the students. They will just send me receipts for their donations because they said it and they thought I would find out. One graduate, Susan H, actually sent me a receipt because she *thought*, "Poor Baby"!

But the point is to catch ourselves, and to be aware that when an animal is vulnerable, we want to protect them emotionally and see them as able to heal or able to be independent or confident.

I charge half, only ten dollars for "Bless his little heart" because that is an American—particularly southern cultural—saying that isn't as bad.

Then we started charging twenty dollars for unsolicited advice. I'm thinking all of the sanctuaries, rescues, and shelters could get rich. Imagine all of the people telling you what to do when you didn't ask?! But that's another story entirely for a healing book!

More Stories

Caden

Years ago, someone gifted a woman, Deidre, with an animal communication session for a beautiful Welsh Pony named Caden. I was pretty sure Deidre didn't believe in animal communication; I could smell the eye roll through the phone. Caden was in full-time training to drive (pull a cart). It wasn't going as well as Deidre had hoped. I could tell from my own intuition that Deidre was a very fair and loving trainer. So, this was important to her, even if she didn't believe in animal communication.

Deirdre sat very stoically waiting to hear what the pony had to say. Through the animal communication session, Caden shared he had a great work ethic, but he needed a longer warm up. He had a tough time engaging with the work because he had always been a late bloomer. He loved his original person and he had gone through a lot emotionally in this transition. He respected Deidre and knew she was in a true struggle to keep him. Apparently, she had lost a lot of clients recently and was struggling financially.

Caden shared that he knew he had armor. He shared that he knew he was distant. He had truly loved someone before. There was someone in between the original person and Deidre that had dismissed him, and he was at the bottom of her priority list. Deep in his heart, he knew and had heard that he came from excellent breeding and was supposed to be something great. But something had gone wrong. Really, wrong.

That's when Deirdre stopped me. She admitted that she hadn't believed in animal communication until that moment. In Deidre's shock, she shared that her friend Sharon had bought the pony sight unseen and expected him to be this great breeding pony because he had won all sorts of awards. When he got off the trailer, he was underdeveloped and skinny. The woman freaked out and demanded her money back for the "goat she bought."

Of course, Sharon never got her money back. While Caden did have the good bloodlines, Sharon never did anything with him, so he sat there in her yard, for years while she stewed and stayed mad at him and the situation. Eventually, Deidre took him on.

Deidre realized that there was so much emotional pain with the pony. There had to be forgiveness. She recognized immediately that Sharon's anger was still zapping his energy. Deidre's momentary enlightenment shifted the situation drastically through her deep compassion. She was able to work with Sharon for forgiveness and Caden excelled in Deidre's program.

Invisibility in Shelters, Rescues, and Sanctuaries

When an animal is in between homes, presumably in a shelter or a rescue, who they truly are—essence or personality—often gets lost in the mix. They are so busy assessing the situation, they aren't exhibiting their true self. Their essence and favorite things get lost in the mix. They become someone we can project onto and often, not accurately. All the things they identified with or the things, people, and places that they knew to be true are just gone. Gone.

Merlin

Merlin was a greyhound who was at a big greyhound rescue. He was being fostered by Louise and her husband Al. They had many other greyhounds, and Louise was on the board of the rescue. They knew greyhounds. As sad and hard as it was for Louise to admit defeat, she was about to return Merlin to the shelter if something wasn't revealed to her in our upcoming animal communication session. In fact, she thought he had lost the will to live.

While nobody loves the world of dog racing, some dogs are treated well and do enjoy their job. Merlin was one of them. He shared with me that he was absolutely spoiled rotten with his original people. He won everything. He was a rock star among greyhounds. And humans!

But here he was in this household with these boring, normal greyhounds. They hadn't had the illustrious career, the excitement, the notoriety. He was casting his pearls before swine. They were beneath him.

As I shared this story with Louise, you could see Merlin rise from the bed he was on as if to say "See, I'm someone. I'm someone great." From that moment forward, Louise and her husband truly saw Merlin for who he was. In his pack, Merlin was highly regarded and lived a very happy life.

THE FOURTH CHAKRA— HEART

"The Heart Chakra is the fourth level of consciousness in the chakra system. It is the home of wisdom, joy, love and compassion for the self and others, and true acceptance of every aspect of ourselves - every impulse, every mistake, every less than perfect part of us. Located smack dab in the middle of the chakras, the Heart Chakra is positioned to deliver lower-chakra energy straight through to the top chakra, or crown chakra. An open heart, when fueled by the lower three chakras, can move mountains in our lives and the lives of those we touch. Here's where we can truly feel empowered."

—MARGARET LYNCH RANIERE and DAVID RANIERE, PH.D.,
Unblocked: A Revolutionary Approach to Tapping into Your Chakra Empowerment Energy to Reclaim Your Passion, Joy, and Confidence

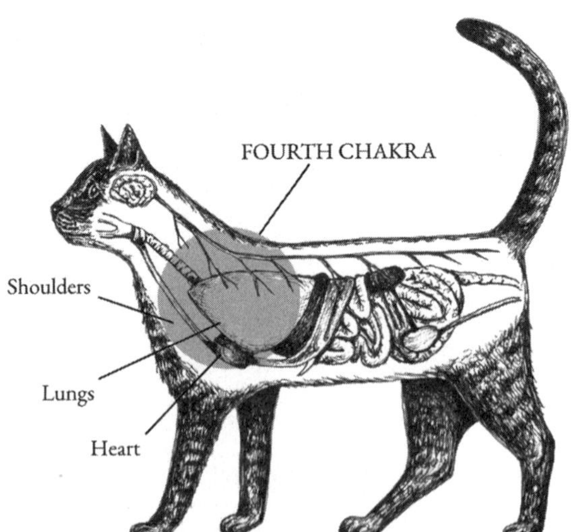

Fig. 5: The fourth chakra (heart chakra)

Big Hearts—Built for Speed

Cheetahs, greyhounds, and thoroughbred horses . . . what do they have in common? They all have the deep thoracic cage to cradle giant hearts, literally, figuratively, and energetically. Those giant hearts are supported by oversized livers, adrenals, lungs, arteries, and bronchi so that the body can explode with speed. They can all jump into a lightning-fast sprint with the blink of an eye. In the case of the thoroughbred, who is prey, that heart and its accompanying organs and glands activate their stride into God-speed.

Cheetahs with their narrow waist and deep chest are the fastest land animals and one of the most endangered species. Their nostrils and lungs are bigger than most cats and their ability to circulate oxygen at high speeds is matched by no other cat. Their tail acts as a rudder in tandem with their flexible spine. The black tear stripe from their eye to their mouth works like a rifle scope so the sun doesn't get in their eyes when they focus on the horizon. The cheetah paw pad has treads built in so that they can make parkour moves in any terrain.

Throughout history, cheetahs have been trapped and tamed. They were trained to ride on the back of a horse to hunt on behalf of the human. The Sumerians were the first to train cheetahs, and the ancient Persians, Egyptians, and Indians followed suit.

Emperor Akbar of India trained over one thousand pet cheetahs for hunting. It was truly a royal sport to hunt with your cheetah. Cheetahs also became pets for many cultures. They have a playful, affable nature and aren't likely to hurt a human unless they are truly threatened.

Cheetahs are associated with elegance, speed, and royalty. In some African tribes, cheetahs are symbolic of justice, focus, speed, determination and, in some cultures, even the swiftness to enlightenment. Kings, pharaohs, and emperors have owned them as a sign of wealth.

Greyhounds were bred for royalty. Literally. Originally from Egypt and Syria, greyhounds have been spoken of in the Quran, the Bible, and both Roman and Greek mythology. They are the oldest purebred dog dating back to the pharaohs. They are the original sighthounds. All sighthounds have descended from the greyhound. Sighthound means that they hunt by sight versus scent.

They too have narrow waists and deep chests. They have long faces, larger lungs, and hearts, built for speed. They are slight with a flexible spine and long legs. They are muscular machines of speed.

They were once used by nomadic tribes to run down game animals. In the Middle Ages, there was an extreme famine that wiped out most dog breeds. The clergy saved the remaining greyhounds and that is how they became the dogs of the aristocracy.

Kings and noblemen made laws against the commoners, preventing them from having greyhounds as they were used for sport—at that time hunting was sport in royal circles. Greyhounds were used for coursing, racing, and hunting. Racing has become their "sport" in modern times.

Greyhounds were once seen as gods. They are equated with noble nature, speed, elegance, determination, strength, and freedom.

Horses were also bred for royalty. Even today, horse racing is considered "the sport of kings."

Thoroughbreds are agile, spirited—meaning hot, hot, hot—and fast. They have been selectively bred from an original stock of 43 mares—Arabians and Barb horses—around the third century. Their breeding was for racing and jumping. They were introduced to the United States around the nineteenth century.

Here in the US, they are primarily bred for racing. That deep barrel with slim legs, sleek neck, and short back was built for speed. They were also used to "improve the breeding" of other known breeds.

Once thoroughbreds are used up by the race industry, if they are lucky, they move into loving homes. These versatile, off-the-track thoroughbreds (OTTB) can have a second career as a jumper, a three-day eventer, dressage horse, or they can have the luxury of being a companion to humans and other horses.

Sadly, this is not the case for many of these horses. And we will uncover that dirty secret in the shadow side below.

Secretariat, the racehorse who won the Triple Crown in 1973, had a heart three times the size of that of a normal horse. Its weight was 22 pounds. The Triple Crown consists of three races: the Kentucky Derby, Preakness Stakes, and Belmont Stakes. Secretariat's running time in each of these races has never been defeated.

Thoroughbreds symbolize speed, elegance, determination, and a free nature that cannot be tamed.

There are other breeds of horses who have similar confirmation, like standardbreds, who actually have a longer back and are heavier boned. They are used for "pacing," a trot race pulling a two-wheel cart. This involves endurance and strategy.

The quarter horse is smaller in size and is known for being able to run a quarter of a mile faster than any other horse.

Both of those breeds have a lot of thoroughbred (big hearts) bred into them.

Of course, the Arabians raced, they have different confirmation, and would be bred for endurance, long-distance running.

And horse racing, bareback or with a chariot, dates to the original Olympics. As a side note, women could compete.

Back to the Heart of the Matter

What can we learn from this and what does it have to do with these giant hearts? How did we come to walk alongside each of these beings? The cheetah has had a big history of walking with humans and of hunting with humans. The greyhound—how did we tame them enough to partner with them? The thoroughbred, how did we still that wild heartbeat enough to slip onto that back and go for speed?

It comes down to not just the size of that heart but its capacity to love and willingness to please.

These animals love fiercely, play with determination, are efficient with their energy, and know when to rest. Let's look deeper into the heart chakra and see what we can glean from those big hearts.

Fourth Chakra Symbolism

The heart chakra is known for being the bridge between the manifest world and the unseen.

The heart chakra poses as a paradox in that together it is a container for:

- Self-love and romantic love
- Sorrow and joy
- Compassion and discernment
- Forgiveness and acceptance
- Grief and peace

And of course, openness, empathy, connection, unconditional love, trust, willingness, and transformation.

In many ways, we could say, it is the center for integration.

The heart chakra is the bridge between our survival and our connection to the divine.

It is also the bridge between the animal kingdom and humans.

When we walk with animals, we walk next to their shoulder, the heart chakra. We walk with our first chakra (our legs) in alignment with their shoulder or forward. Think of the element of trust and willingness they must have to allow our survival center to lead their hearts!

Fourth Chakra Species-Specific/Wild and Domestic

For the most part, for most animals, the size of the heart is a fraction of their actual size. I love to geek out on weird wildlife facts, so I thought I would share. Some have unusual hearts, some hearts enable great speeds, and the rest are just huge hearts. While we don't walk along beside these wild animals and their heart chakra, we definitely open our hearts with childlike wonder to them.

Did you know …

Big hearts:

- Blue whales: their heart weighs 440 pounds!
- African elephants have giant hearts to fill in and support that big body. And, to love and nurture their extended family.
- Manatee, it doesn't take a biologist to discover this. Manatees are all heart!

Unique hearts:

- Crocodiles have an extra "hole" or valve from the heart to the stomach that pumps blood and carbon dioxide to help it digest big meals.
- Zebra fish have unusual heart cells that can regenerate heart tissue after extensive damage.

- And while we're in the sea, did you know that an octopus has three hearts!
- The emperor penguin has a diving heart rate way slower than it's resting heart rate, which helps them to circulate oxygen and stay in frigid temperatures for up to 18 minutes!
- Of course, the dog has the highest heart-to-body ratio.

Speed

Some animals are just built for speed, and the big heart is part of that equation.

If you've ever been outside and chased by a horsefly, you won't be surprised to find out that they can fly up to 90 mph!

But the peregrine falcon has the horsefly beat. Peregrine falcons have been clocked in midair dives at 200 to 240 mph. WOW. They have an aerodynamic build, kind of like the cheetah, the greyhound, and the thoroughbred. And they have a very long wingspan, enabling them to fly long distances. They tuck in their wings when they dive through the air. You will find that wings are part of the heart chakra when we get to the anatomy part of this chapter.

Wildebeest have a deep barrel for a big heart, and they claim speed as a superpower.

Springbok might be the fastest antelope, with an impressive top speed of 55 mph.

Dragonflies can travel at 30 mph—crazy!

Black Marlin are the fastest fish, coming in at 80 mph!

The Shadow Side of the Fourth Chakra

In this chakra, we will explore the individual's shadow side with this chakra, and what happens in certain "industries" because of big-hearted, good-willed animals.

In other words, that very thing we love, that very thing we need, that very thing we honor:

Speed, elegance, determination, and a free nature that cannot be tamed.

This could be applied to all three: cheetahs (the most endangered); greyhounds (one of the most exploited dog breeds); and thoroughbreds (one of the most exploited horse breeds)—and it is all because of their giant heart.

It could also be applied to every other big-hearted animal, regardless of breed or species.

Cheetahs and other big cats are often seen as a status symbol and are still "owned" by people. People believe, *If I can handle this animal, I can handle anything.*

The human–wildlife conflict is a big portion of an animal's endangerment but also animal trafficking, owning and/or killing wildlife for individual needs.

In the center of Kuwait City, psychologist Adnan al-Shatti intimately knows the fears, phobias, and eccentric hobbies of his fellow countrymen: "A lot of people here like challenges, and they do not want a classic pet, but an extraordinary animal that resists them," Shatti says. "This is also about looking different from ordinary people. If I can deal with such an animal, it means that I'm superior," he adds.

"In Kuwait, there is also a culture of non-regulation. In the conscience, there is no barrier. Everything is possible if we have money."

Greyhound racing is now illegal in 42 states. Hopefully, it is on the way out. That said, like horse racing, I've connected and communicated with many, many greyhounds who have been proud of their work and loved their people.

Most of their lives, these social creatures spend their time alone, living in cramped crates and small, fenced enclosures for 20 to 23 hours a day. They could have injuries that go unattended. Every three days, a greyhound dies at the track in Florida.

The horseracing industry is known for its cruelty. Again, a racehorse may have a great experience. Often, they are treated so well and have fancier lives than most humans. They also pay for it as their body breaks down as they are sent to work when they are underdeveloped, young, full-of-energy animals who should be out playing in a field together. They are put in a tough regimen and often fed less than perfect food. Their meals would consist of highly acidic, oversaturated sugary grains to promote big bursts of energy to make those mile-long sprints. They are over-vaccinated and ingest a lot of chemical wormers. Their young bodies are so taxed by the time that they retire at age three or four, that they then break down rather regularly in their next careers.

If I had a dime for every time I have seen a beautiful horse who had been imported from Europe only to come to the States and break down, I'd have a lot of money. The horses who are willing, sensitive, and athletic get pushed too hard, live under too much pressure and they often break, either mentally or physically.

Sometimes when we walk side by side with them, as humans we tend to exploit that very thing we love about them, or their very instinct. This is true of, for example, their natural tendency for healthy competition born out of fun and youthful activity. The same could be said for dogs in the agility ring or the racing industry.

- Horses who are so willing to please end up being broken down early.
- Dogs have similar experiences to horses.
- Overvaccination, chemical worming, and foods that produce too much "heat" to make horses hot at the track have an adverse effect on the immune system moving forward.
- Chronic front-end lameness is a widespread issue in these arenas.

Other animals whose good natures and big hearts get exploited:

- Beagles' great, sweet nature gets taken advantage of because of our need for animal testing.
- Big-hearted mama cows have to give up their babies so that they can produce milk for human consumption. The babies are kept nearby, crying for their mamas, so that the hormones course through the mama's grieving, helpless body, and the milk flows for the baby around the corner. That baby, if it is a girl, will never see the milk but will be raised on hormones for the same fate as her mother. The baby boy will never see the light of day as he becomes veal.
- Along the same lines as the docile loving cows, the "nurse mare" industry for racehorses is appalling. The thoroughbred racehorses who have been bred but must get back to work, have to give up their foals, who then get put on a nurse mare or "junk mare." What does that mean? The nurse mare nurses the foal. The only way for a nurse mare to have milk is if she just had a foal. Her foal gets left behind. Often dying from neglect.

Fourth Chakra Organs, Structure, Body Parts, and Meridians

Organs

The fourth chakra is green. Healing, delicious green. Physically, this chakra governs our heart, pericardium, lungs, bronchial tubes, upper back, shoulders, wings, pectoral fins, and breasts. The rib cage houses and protects those organs, which are very tender, emotional in nature, and life affirming.

- Physiological systems at work here: respiratory (inhales oxygen, exhales unwanted carbon dioxide), cardiovascular (blood flow), and circulatory (carries blood to and away from heart).
- Endocrine systems at work here: Thymus.
- Nerve plexus: Cardiac plexus, speaks to the autonomic system and ganglia at the base of the heart—both sympathetic and parasympathetic nervous systems, peripheral nervous system (PNS).
- Spine: Thoracic T1-T12.
- BONUS in the Heart Chakra: The thoracic sling, which is basically a muscle group that literally acts like a sling to hold up the chest between the front limbs.

Meridians and Traditional Chinese Medicine

Conception Vessel (CV), Governing Vessel (GV), Lungs (LU), Large Intestine (LI), Stomach (ST), Spleen/Pancreas (SP), Heart (HE), Small Intestine (SI), Pericardium (PC), Triple Heater (TH), and Gallbladder (GB).

The lung meridian (yin) starts on the inside of the chest area and comes front paw or hoof up to the inside of the chest.

The large intestine (yang) starts on the front of the paw or hoof and comes up the front legs, through the neck, and up to the nose.

The spleen meridian (yin) starts on the fourth toe, or dew claw, or at the second toe on the hind foot, and travels up the inside of the hind legs, across the bottom of the torso, up to the area that would be like an armpit, and then toward the withers. It connects on the hind feet with its yang (masculine) counterpart, the stomach.

The pericardium meridian (yin) is on the inside of the front legs, meeting up at the chest, where it also meets the kidney meridian. The pericardium is the thin layer that protects the heart. This meridian has an energetic component in that it is the literal and energetic protector of the heart. The pericardium meridian is used to promote joy.

The triple heater (yang) starts on the front of the front paw or hoof, goes up the front of the leg, up the shoulder, up the neck, over the top of the ear, and down to the outside of the eyes. This meridian is not associated with an organ. Just as it suggests, the triple heater (along with the kidney meridian) is responsible for metabolism and regulating the entire system.

Putting It All together: The Rib Cage

The rib cage houses and protects those organs, which are very tender. Each of the organs seem to be the most emotional in nature, and life-affirming. Some of the challenges related to the heart chakra:

- Breast cancer
- Heart murmurs
- Asthma
- Allergies
- Heart disease
- Lung challenges
- Congestive heart failure
- Lung cancer
- Pneumonia
- High blood pressure

- This area gets sore and breaks down when the animal has a weak hind end; it becomes part of a pattern to compensate for that weakness. The shoulders and necks of dogs that have lost the use of their hind ends can be rock hard, like armor. These are the dogs that carry the world on their shoulders.
- In horses, an ill-fitting saddle at the withers (the ridge between the shoulders on four-legged animals) is very common. Continuing the theme of horses having many homes and many jobs, this area is very susceptible to saddle challenges.
- Many horses that have had a hind end injury will compensate by overdoing it on the forehand (front end).
- Birds with clipped wings lose their ability for exercise thus contributing to less circulation and more hormonal and mental health issues.

Margaret Lynch calls this chakra " . . . the great integrator of the true self. It is capable of bringing all the chakras together to make us feel whole." I feel like it is also the great integrator of the human/animal relationship. Like unseen connective tissue.

Fourth Chakra Emotions and Energetics

In many ways, the heart center holds the paradox of the being, at times a great contradiction. We can see this as it welcomes all the emotions.

This area governs emotional expression, love, romantic love, unconditional love, and universal love. The heart center is the home of joy. It also holds hopes and dreams. The heart center is the home of forgiveness. We can see an open-hearted animal from a mile away. We can also see, feel, and experience the shutdown of an animal. Often, they will have a lot of armor around their broken heart.

It is the epicenter of unbridled passion, unending affection, a burst of anger, and the ability to nurture others. We see those cats who will nurse orphan kittens, or a chicken who will take on a duckling.

In human terms, maturity is the ability to hold sorrow and joy at the same time. In many ways our animals exemplify this as they navigate moment by moment. They could have had a big loss and feel it deep in their hearts, moping around, yet, they can still exude joy when a visitor comes over.

Those emotions and sensations are:

- Heartfelt compassion
- Compassion for self
- Self-acceptance
- Unconditional love
- Neutral
- Wisdom
- Joy
- Grief
- Rage
- Panic
- Fear
- Bravery
- Hope
- Pride
- Anticipation
- Expectation
- Disappointment
- Defeat
- Content
- Willingness
- Devotion
- Loyalty
- Curiosity
- Childlike wonder

The fourth chakra can house a broken heart and be a great space for healing it. We can channel our inner zebra fish!

So many animals "shoulder" the world. We see animals who literally die of a broken heart. And often animals who have had so many homes have a wall of protection around their heart center. It can be quite apparent in the lack of interest with the world or even big bulky shoulder and a deep chest cavity.

Horses may have challenges in the heart center, due to an ill-fitting saddle, the withers—the ridge between the shoulders on four-legged animals—will be very tight and sometimes damaged.

Sometimes horses and dogs have had many jobs, and either haven't experienced full satisfaction, or haven't been acknowledged for their work or contribution.

Cats can often be the unnoticed—big—heart of the household. When their "contribution" of love or overseeing the emotion of the household goes unnoticed, this can often be connected to litterbox issues.

The Essence

In my teachings in either books or the school, Communication with all Life University, we start all animal communication with understanding what the "essence" of the animal is—with whom we are communicating. The essence of an animal is how its persona shows up. I also sometimes refer to it as the archetype that the animal embodies. If you think of the soul as a continuum among all beings, the essence is how the soul shows up in this species and this individual animal in this lifetime.

Looking for the animal's essence is a way to deepen your connection. Appreciating and acknowledging the animal's personality quirks gives you good information about their behavior, their purpose, and any jobs they may want to do as well. It also provides insight into what might be helpful in any healing process.

The essence is fluid and evolving. Nobody is ever one thing. The essence helps to define the animal's character and qualities: Is he a mama's boy? The baby girl? Is she independent and aloof? Would you consider him/her to be a teacher? A healer? A familiar? A lover? A nurturer? A partner? A twin flame? From another realm like the fairy kingdom, the angelic realm, or a spirit guide? And ultimately, that heart dog/cat/horse or soulmate.

In ancient Egypt it was believed that the heart center was the seat of the soul. Some believe it is in the eighth chakra, more on that later.

Many of us know what it is to have a soulmate animal. Many of us know what it is to have a heart animal. People will say this is my heart dog, or my heart cat, or my heart horse.

What is the difference between a soulmate and a heartmate?

A soulmate animal is one animal that speaks to your soul and has seemingly been with you for lifetimes. It's deep. It has no beginning or no end. It's like a partnership that has no words. These animals leave a giant hole in our heart when they leave.

A heart dog, heart horse or heart cat speaks to the heart. They spark a certain joy, and hope. When something happens to them, we dive into a place where disappointment could come in so deeply that it hurts our heart.

And do you have to only have one? Absolutely not. The greatest thing about soulmate or heartmate animals is that we don't have to be monogamous.

Fourth Chakra Behavior, Dynamics, and Relationships

Often, we can feel the heartbeat of another. Riders feel the heartbeat of the horse. After a big spook, or encountering something scary, a rider may feel that big heartbeat for a while. The rider will feel the heart rate slow, and the adrenalin melt away as you walk on.

My cat got out this morning and under that thick blanket of tabby fur I could see a boom-boom, boom-boom as he sniffed the air. In his crouched curiosity, his heartbeat was visible.

We can feel their heartbeat through the leash before the dog raises his head or positions him/herself. It's like the nostrils are in sync with the heartbeat, and vice versa. When we come upon that dog who attacked us or see a dog in the distance, knowing that our dog is a big ole attack dog wannabe, and our shirt starts bopping to the unusual heart rate, and you know it wasn't caffeine. Yes, your dog feels that before you say, "Hey, let's go the other direction."

It's hard to say whose heartbeat starts the blast-off.

And it's not just fear that is revealed through the heartbeat. In many shows or trials, you can see the person and their dog as they lift off through the agility jumps or that fluid dressage ride. In competition, you can't say "good boy," "good girl," or "good job." Rather, you feel the contentment of the heart, as if the heart is smiling.

We feel this in our homes.

Stories

Isis and Zeus

Isis and Zeus were two magnificent German shepherds who were as in love with each other, as they were with their human, Gina. They were truly soulmates. Zeus suddenly died of a heart attack at the age of nine. Gina felt robbed, and Isis was inconsolable.

Gina was in a divorce. Zeus was more her soulmate than her husband had ever been.

Through an animal communication session, Isis revealed that Zeus was her soulmate.

Between Gina and Isis, the household was smothering with grief. The little dog Betty revealed to me that she could hardly breathe. The grief was an impenetrable wall. Isis could barely get out of her dog bed and Gina was limping along through life, pulling her broken heart around like a rickety wagon.

I did EFT (Emotional Freedom Technique) Tapping sessions, with both Gina and Isis. The next day, Gina sent me a video. Gina shared that she heard a weird noise and went outside. It turns out that the weird noise was Betty and Isis leaping through the doggy door. When Gina went outside, she found Betty chasing Isis, and Isis turning around and chasing Betty. Gina made a video as she stood in astonishment. The glee on the dogs' faces of finding fun again was infectious.

While both Gina and Isis missed Zeus terribly and largely had to redefine their lives without him, they found joy again, and fun with Betty.

Healing All the Broken Hearts

Mole is a giant personality only slightly contained in a Chihuahua body. He suddenly seized up and when Val got him to the hospital, it was discovered that he had a tear in his heart and that there was fluid surrounding the heart. The prognosis wasn't good. The vets could drain the fluid around the heart but had no way of doing anything more than that. It was basically take him home and wait for his next episode, or the expected decline.

The truth is that the home had been broken up. Val's husband, Adam, had left in a temporary separation. Val was heartbroken. Their teenage daughter may not have admitted to heartbreak, and she may have enjoyed the extra mommy time, but the disappointment was deep. Adam was heartbroken. When he got the initial distress call from Val, he met her at the hospital for the diagnosis. In defeat, he went back home with Val to be with Mole in what they thought were his last hours.

Adam decided to stay, and love was in repair.

And Mole is still among us upon typing this. He is a slightly muted version of his big badass self in a little body. With a heart repaired by love.

Jeff and Freedom

Because I do the work I do, I have the privilege and honor to meet so many wonderful animals and their people. Some of the stories are so extraordinary and one of the greatest stories I've ever heard is the story of Jeff and Freedom.

I used to get this email rather regularly about a guy who saved an eagle baby and then the baby lived and helped him through cancer. It has a picture of a guy and an eagle. Somewhere it said the guy's name and the eagle's name. I looked this story up on Snopes (back in the day, this was a website that dispels urban myths). Sure enough, as I looked this amazing story up, not only was it true, but the guy also had a book out called *An Eagle Named Freedom: My True Story of a Remarkable Friendship*. His name is Jeff Guidry, and he was about to have a book signing in Seattle on the next day. I was forty-five minutes out of the city so I decided that I would attend the signing.

So, I found him on Facebook, we were friends instantly, and he noticed I lived in the next town over from him. I went to the book signing, I had him on my-then radio show and we became fast friends. In no time, I was invited to visit Freedom the Eagle.

Jeff's book tells the story of Freedom, how she was a little three-month-old baby eagle who was injured so severely that she'd never go back to the wild. He had connected with her, but she was touch and go as she wouldn't stand up in her cage. She was very depressed. Jeff was beside himself. Finally on the day she was to be euthanized, Jeff discovered that she was standing just for him.

After recovering with pins in one wing, she became part of the educational program at Sarvey Wildlife Center. Jeff and eagle travel together and she helps people to understand something about eagles.

There is also something beyond majestic, preternatural about her—you could say that she has an otherworldly angelic presence.

Because of that, when Jeff was diagnosed with Hodgkin's lymphoma, Freedom was Jeff's solace. It goes even further than that though; when Jeff was asleep, he would dream of Freedom flying in and eating the cancer out of his system. Jeff went through chemo yet truly considers Freedom his healer. Jeff has been symptom free for some time now.

To stand in the presence of greatness is humbling. I would have to say that anyone who has met Freedom experiences that. Jeff has to go to great lengths to protect her because people do project onto her that she can heal.

It is a presence of the wild, the proud, and overcoming great obstacles. There just aren't words to describe it. She has chosen to stay here to teach—to be in her presence requires being present. When I take my Animal Communication classes up there to meet her, they are overwhelmed. Usually everyone is a little teary eyed, and words fail us. And it's the love, the love and the beauty and the grace she exudes. She reaches a part of our soul that wants to be all that she is.

I asked Jeff what it is that he thought she gave to people. He told me, "Confidence. She puts them in touch with their own inner strength. I tell people she's not healing. Her presence changes us because we are in awe of this presence. You forget your troubles. With the concrete we keep losing our connection. We lose the essence of the wild. She reminds everybody – hey! We're here!"

Fooey

I share a story in my book, *Emotional Freedom Technique for Animals and Their Humans* about Shakespeare, the horse that got me tapping on a horse to begin with. Shakespeare had an epic fear of ponies and became blindly aggressive toward them. I had been using the tapping techniques on humans for a while, for say, if they had a horse accident. or a reactive dog, but Shakespeare made me do it. I tapped on a horse. Because I knew tapping AND acupressure, I was able to have amazing success.

His person, Joanne, had another horse. Fooey. Fooey was a giant—and I mean giant—chocolate morsel. He was just drop dead gorgeous and huge, but he had been dumped several times and Joanne didn't know what to do with him. She just wasn't connecting with him.

On top of it all, at a dinner party on a Saturday night, Joanne announced that she was going to euthanize Fooey because she couldn't get on top of his wicked sinus infection since she purchased him a year ago and antibiotics weren't touching it. Joanne felt that his immune system was so compromised after a year-long infection, there was no way his immune system could fight it at this point. Our mutual friend and horse trainer and I shot a glance at each other and then I stood up. "Give me a week."

So, it began. On Monday morning, I was there with my Rife Machine, a profound healing mechanism. But in my twenty-two years with this same machine, I have found that tweaking the codes with energy work is what works best. The Rife Machine was created by Dr. Royal Rife, who believed that all cancer had an underlying parasite and possibly a bacteria/virus/candida accompanying the parasites. The frequency codes address and activate healing on one of those levels. All modern-day cold lasers that veterinarians are using now are based on the original codes of Dr. Royal Rife.

While the machine worked on the infection, I worked on the grief. And when I say buckets of snot came out, I mean buckets of snot came out. We literally filled buckets in the fancy barn aisle as I stood on a ladder and worked on this fine fellow. He was ready and willing to release all his grief, all of his uncried tears. He was ready to be someone's number one.

Fooey had always been number two to someone and now he was number two to Shakespeare. Shakespeare was Joanne's number one guy. Fooey was too polite to put up a fight, but he internalized this in his lungs and sinuses. He was never going to put up a stink or demand, he just hurt deeply inside.

Fooey knew that he didn't belong on the show circuit, or even in the jumping world, if somebody didn't take his heart and soul into consideration. We did EFT Tapping on all of his disappointment and "failures in humans' eyes."

Fooey had a bit more of a bumpy road to his perfect home, but he ended up being the love and guide of one gal's life. Shelly loved jumping, groundwork with horses, and bodywork. He benefitted from all her passions. She now has a farm sanctuary outside of the Seattle area. Allowing animals to be animals after their healing journey, and her experience with Fooey, were important steps to her understanding the need to create a sanctuary.

Tess and Diane

Tess and Diane are a team known in sheep herding circles. Tess has been a healer for Diane not once but twice and both rather significantly. Diane and her husband had really suffered over a miscarriage and Tess, a gorgeous border collie, came into their lives. Diane didn't have time for her grief after a certain point because Tess was so frightened of things. She had to overdo the training in order to give Tess confidence. A byproduct of Tess overcoming her fear was that Diane overcame her loss.

One summer day, Diane's husband, Getty pulled into the farm that they had just bought and said, "Look honey, I bought you a farm for your birthday." Diane said, "My birthday isn't until next month." Getty said, "Not you, Diane, today is Tessy's birthday." That's how the sheep herding farm began.

Diane is a successful handler and teaches sheep herding. Tess became known as one of the most talented dogs in North America; she was sixth in the nation and the third sheepdog to be registered on merit.

Her real healing job began when Diane had a horse accident and had to have her ribs x-rayed. The doctor discovered that her heart was enlarged, and that the upper chamber was gone; there was no wall between the upper right and left chamber of the heart. She was rushed into open heart surgery, actually two surgeries, in one day. The recovery didn't go well, her lungs filled with blood. She had to have more surgeries and the healing took months longer than anticipated.

Tess very tenuously walked around Diane to not knock her down. She hovered over her and nursed her. If Diane cried in pain, Tess was right there. She stood between anyone and Diane and would growl to protect her.

Diane felt she was going down a very long tunnel, she knew she was dying. It was freeing, no pain, until she felt the very sharp pain of Tess biting her arm and clawing at her. Then the panic-stricken dog sat and licked Diane's face. Eventually, Diane knew that she was truly healing when Tess stopped hovering. Diane calls her the little heart dog and feels that Tess is her healer and teacher.

THE FIFTH CHAKRA—THROAT/GIVING VOICE

"Vishuddha is the center for communicating our truth to the world. It is about giving voice - or music or sound - to our inner heart, and in turn hearing what the world has to reply.

This is the last of the chakras that processes the gross or physical elements. Within its location, we prepare to ascend the ladder of consciousness, to shift into the chakras devoted to spirituality. It is time to ask what needs to be said to make this transcendence possible."

—CYNDI DALE, *The Subtle Body: An Encyclopedia of Your Energetic Anatomy*

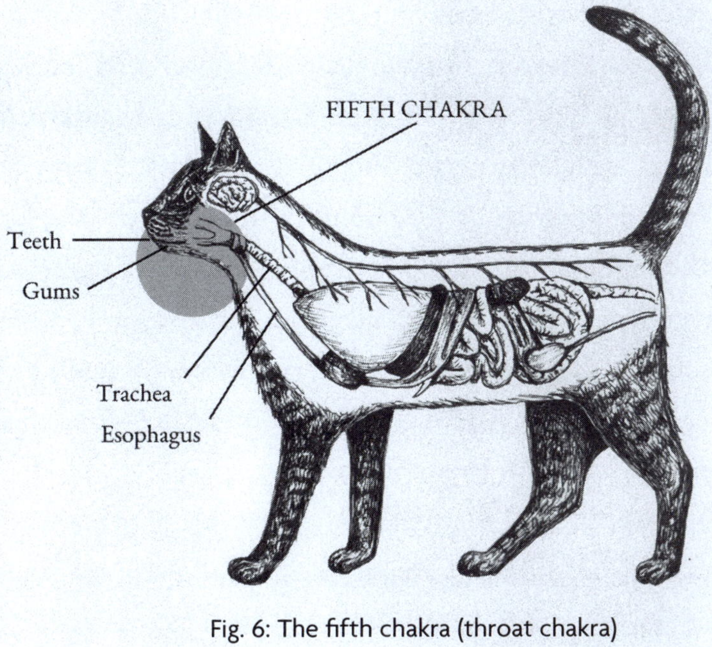

Fig. 6: The fifth chakra (throat chakra)

Express Yourself – All Beings Have a Voice

Every morning, starting at dawn, I can hear the gibbons singing. In fact, throughout the morning, they will rev up the singing engine and let it rip. No, I don't live in a southeast Asian tropical rainforest. I live up the street, well, dirt road, from the Gibbon Conservation Center. When I first moved in, I thought, "Is that a high school pep rally?"

There are roughly 37 gibbons representing about seven of the 20 species of gibbons. In fact, all these different gibbon species expressing themselves is also a sight to see as they swing back and forth in their enclosures. It could be quite a cacophony and, yet, all of those voices ringing through as they seem to search for harmony sound inspiring.

It's like they egg each other on, and the expression becomes more and more profound and individual, while instinctual. It is quite magical.

I've been fortunate enough to have heard gibbons singing in the wild—like a familiar wakeup call around 6 a.m.—when I took people on one of my wildlife trips to Borneo.

In the wild, gibbons are dwindling at a rapid rate. This is tragic for a thousand reasons. Gibbons, by nature, are a bit introverted and stay close with their family, as long as they get along. Yet, they are charismatic acrobats, and their pure expression is released through song.

The gibbon song is meant to determine territory in the dense forests where they originate. It is also a way to get a date! The song lures in the partner and, once established as a pair, they sing a duet that strengthens their bond. Their offspring sing the family song until they are of dating age, and then their song breaks off as they leave their family system.

They find expression built into their day. All beings need to express themselves. Let's look at the fifth chakra, the chakra of expression and communication.

When the pandemic hit and lockdown was in full swing, I had so many New Yorkers tell me that they could hear the birds sing for the very first time.

When I go down to feed horses in the morning with my dogs in tow, I hear a small symphony, as if the birds in this set of trees are the section of flutes and recorders. They harmonize with some oboes and clarinets, and over in this other set of trees we have the bassoon and trumpet and the cows across the street provide a little base cello. It is busy. When the sound isn't melodic, I know it's an alarm cry, and when it's silent, I know there is a predator. As soon as the threat leaves, it's as if someone turned up the volume, and the musical expression continues.

Every place I visit on my wildlife retreats has its own morning soundtrack. To experience the most sightings, we leave early, and I mean early in the morning. While we are looking for bigger animals, the sweet sounds of black-headed orioles and sighting wrens, rollers and hornbills makes life all the softer.

Song almost feels like a portal to heaven, doesn't it?

For seven years I took people on wild dolphin trips. One of the greatest things on earth was to slip into the water and to be able to hear the dolphins in the distance. I almost had to tune my ear to attract that frequency because it could easily go unnoticed.

In 2015, I took a Marine Wildlife Naturalist course through the Whale Museum in Friday Harbor, Washington, studying the marine wildlife, in particular the Orcas surrounding the San Juan Islands in the Salish Sea. I later took another Marine Naturalist course in Orange County, California. These classes are addictive if you like to learn.

One of my most favorite moments was when we put the hydrophones in the water to listen to the whales communicate with each other. In fact, they have a hydrophone you can connect with at Lime Kiln Lighthouse on San Juan Island on the internet. Sometimes you just hear water but at other times you can hear the Orcas cruising through the straights there.

Whales have clicks, whistles, and pulsed calls. We will talk more about clicks and navigation in Chapter 6, when we discuss echolocation and the sixth chakra. The whistles and pulsed calls are more communication and socialization—if you've ever been together with the J, K, and L Superpod when they come together in August of every year, it is more like a party.

Other fun whale facts:

- A humpback whale song can last for over 20 minutes and be heard for over 100 meters.
- A tale slap on the water can get the attention of other whales (and prey) for a very long distance.

Other animals who make sounds range from frogs, crocodilians, geckos, birds, and mammals. The dominant form of communication could be territorial, fright, aggression, alarm, contentment, hunger, presence of food, rage, need for companionship, territorial, mating calls, and even that last sharp cry out for help when facing death. While some of that sounds like a bland laundry list, the expression and communication of animals within their species and within their territory can be as nuanced and prolific as the complexity of each individual.

Expression in Other Forms

Whether it is a horse bolting through the gate and bucking like crazy, or a dog erupting with barking, or a cat who flies through the house after a great poop in the litter box, expression isn't limited to vocalization. When an animal is beaming with joy, proud of something they did, furious and in a rage—all these things are evident through body language and telepathically palpable.

Our own animals express themselves every day. Or they don't, and then we know something is up. Often, when an animal suffers after an injury, surgery, or attack, they must retreat into themselves to conjure up the healing energy or courage necessary to carry on. When we see them disappear on us, that becomes their own form of expression, and we know something is up.

Some cats have a certain purr for the refrigerator and others have a demand meow for "open the door, fool."

Dogs have alert barks, someone is walking down the street bark, I need you to pay attention to me bark. The best new bark I discovered here was "Rattlesnake on the patio bark." My dog Penelope literally created a bark I'd never heard, which got my attention. It was as if the bark had walled off the rattlesnake, which then rattled away, and my cats shot into the house unharmed. That snake was rattling away in full expression because it was threatened and wanted to be left alone.

When we pay attention to the small details it is amazing how specific and important each sound is. And that leads to the communication of this chakra, understanding exactly what they need and want.

Body language is a very clear sign of communication and expression. The dropping of the ears, the tucking of the tail.

In my wildlife trips, guides will often talk about the zones of wildlife. We always try to stay within the safety zone. But this is the order it goes for wildlife:

- Safe zone—the animal continues to graze, play with their babies, or do whatever it was doing, whether it acknowledges your existence or not.

- Too-close zone—we start to see the body stiffen, ears are moving, we might see the whites of the eyes, even hear a snort, a growl, or a roar, often they will seem surprised.
- Threat zone—now the animal is appearing to posture, pose, threaten . . .
- Danger zone—bigger posturing, revving up to . . .
- I-have-to-attack zone.

All without words. And we don't like that. Because we haven't bothered to understand this communication.

It is the very same subtle set of cues our animals in our home give us. But again, like a foreign language we haven't bothered to learn, we are confused by the signals. Then they get punished for something that they were abundantly clear about.

Fifth Chakra Symbolism

The fifth chakra, the throat chakra, is associated with the color blue and has always been considered the center for the voice, the expression, the will. It is about surrendering the will to the hands of God, or the Divine, or the Universe. When activating that universal voice, some would say we are "Speaking the word of God." Caroline Myss even says:

> "Sacred Truth: The fifth chakra is the center of choice and consequence, of spiritual karma. Every choice we make, every thought and feeling we have, is an act of power that has biological, environmental, social, personal, and global consequences. We are everywhere our thoughts are and thus our personal responsibility includes our energy contributions."

She goes on to say:

> "Surrender personal will to Divine will."

In many ways, animals embody this. They are at our will, at our mercy, and yet they have buoyancy and individuation.

Fifth Chakra Species-Specific/Wild and Domestic

My childhood friend Conleth had an African grey parrot named Dillon. When I would call Conleth, I could hear in the background Dillon saying: "Hey Joan." On the one hand, that could be an imitation BUT, when I went over to her house, he would do a literal fly by, saying, "Hey Joan," and even grab my hair.

One spring evening, as the sun was still high in the sky, I was having dinner at Conleth's house. She let Dillon out of his cage, and he waddled over to the table, made his way up the table leg and positioned himself in the perfect place to steal some fresh vegetables from our salad.

Conleth and I were engaged in a story, she was sharing about how she was not paying attention in a situation, and she was jolted into reality. As she was saying, "It was one of those Earth to Conleth moments," Dillon started laughing out loud. So of course, we started laughing and kept repeating "Earth to Conleth," which made Dillon laugh more—and we were crying we were laughing so hard. A truly magical combination of Dillon's complete understanding of the moment conceptually, and exactly who Conleth is!

It reminds me so much of one of my favorite books, *Alex & Me: How a Scientist and a Parrot Discovered a Hidden World of Animal Intelligence—and Formed a Deep Bond in the Process* by Irene M. Pepperberg (HarperCollins, 2009).

Throughout the book, Irene M. Pepperberg, a psychologist, worked closely and became best friends with Alex, an African grey, who not only proved that he understood language and could communicate, but that he also actually understood complex ideas. They had a love for each other like no other. Every night that she left the laboratory, he said: "You be good, I love you."

After his death, in the book, Pepperberg says:

> "Scientifically speaking, the single greatest lesson Alex taught me, taught all of us, is that animal minds are a great deal more like human minds than the vast majority of behavioral scientists believed—or, more importantly, were even prepared to concede might be remotely possible. Now, I am not saying that animals are miniature humans with somewhat lower-octane mental powers, although when Alex strutted around the lab and gave orders to all and sundry, he gave the appearance of being a feathery Napoleon. Yet animals are far more than the mindless automatons that mainstream science held them to be for so long. Alex taught us how little we know about animal minds and how much more there is to discover. This insight has profound implications, philosophically, sociologically, and practically. It affects our view of the species Homo sapiens and its place in nature."

While I abhor animal testing, and animals in laboratories, this book is my one exception. Everyone would fall in love with Alex and all his quirky behaviors and ugly cry upon his death like I did. *Alex & Me* describes relationship and communication on such a profound level in a way that each of you reading this book have not only experienced but craved—having that kind of transparency and connectivity with all life, all of the time.

And I know I fell into the super lucky club. I have spent almost half of my life making a living helping people with that connection. Animal communication is a gateway for people and animals to have a better, deeper relationship, and/or understanding of why their animal was acting in such a way. I used to say that my day job was as an animal communicator but clearly, I was an animal/human counselor! Through telepathic communication, relationships improved with people and their animals, or between the animals in their household.

Sometimes my work has included zoos. Like laboratory testing, horse racing, and several other industries I don't love, these animals still deserve to have a voice, so I always said yes to helping them.

The level of communication I see on my wildlife trips is amazing. So many species are communicating within their species and with other species, all the time—and work together in symbiotic relation to and with each other.

I've been deep in the Bwindi Impenetrable Forest National Park in Uganda trekking up a mountainside to see the Rushegura gorilla family. The trekking guides can emit the "everything is cool" signal by doing the "belch" vocalization, which is a very guttural sound to the silverback, the lead male. The next thing we know, we are within smelling distance of these magnificent creatures, and all is well. The big gorilla daddy continues to play with his grandchildren and my jaw is left on the ground as I'm awestruck at the joy.

I've been so close to lions and had such a sense of peace. One of those times in Hwange National Park in Zimbabwe, several feet away from a pride of lions, two adult females, and lots of babies bouncing around. There was a bushy barrier, so I repositioned myself to be able to see the wild play of the babies between the leaves. In an instant, one of the mama's head popped up and she shot a stern glance my way, and a low growl. It was sharp and quick. I sat back down as if Mother Superior had slapped my hand to tell me just how things are going to be in the second grade. With an energetic dunce cap on, I verbally and vocally apologized profusely. She laid her head back down undramatically to nap and I felt the peace restored immediately.

It's in experiences such as these when we experience not only vocalized communication, but also the feeling or concept is conveyed. On each of my wildlife trips, I lead lots of meditations so that we come to the animals in peace and appreciation. As a result, my groups and I always have experiences that can't be replicated or explained. Even though many of the people on the trips are not "communicators" or haven't done my programs, they feel, sense, and experience who these beings are because of all the forms of communication going on.

Back to Communication and Vocalization

I think a fascinating part of the vocalized communication in vertebrates ranging from mammal to bird to fish to frog is that all the beings have a choana, a posterior nasal cavity with two openings. To make intentional communication—not just sounds—communication requires the respiratory system to be fully engaged and integrated in the delivery of sound. A vocalization is fully realized with a deep breath in, and a push of air up out of the lungs.

Baleen whales don't have vocal cords, instead their airwaves push the tissue between a cushion of fat and muscle. With massive amounts of air, they can create elaborate songs with no "voice box."

These are intentional vocalizations as a form of communication. How many animals emit a frequency we can't even hear? And of course, there is vibrational communication like fungi networks, or the root system of plants, and trees, or even elephants connecting with far away family members through the earth.

The Shadow Side of the Fifth Chakra

We can go on about the beauty and enlightenment of communication, but the burning truth is, we haven't listened. The overarching, overlighting theme of every animal's life is that they haven't had a voice. In the US, they weren't even recognized as sentient until 1976. The European Union finally recognized them as sentient in 1997.

French philosopher, René Descartes considered animals "material automata," lacking souls or consciousness, and incapable of feelings or suffering. This anthropocentric view had taken hold long before Descartes.

Religion and science have had good cause to keep this perspective. Otherwise . . . the screams of torture would be heard loud and clear, whether it be their last breath on the high priests' chopping block as the baby Lamb being sacrificed was for the "common good," or whether it would be the bunny losing an eye to see if mascara is chemically balanced, or whether it's mustangs being torn from their families in roundups.

Even though evolution only caught up to animal consciousness in 1927, there were plenty of "us" types who always knew, regardless of what science or religion preached about it, that animals have souls. Animals have thoughts, feelings, a self-awareness, they have a history, a future, they have karma, wounding, experiences to work through, they have a trajectory, they have purpose, and a mission.

They need agency.

There were other whole cultures who saw this as well.

Animism is the oldest known belief system in the world. Animals, plants, weather systems, rocks, river systems, buildings, and thought forms have life, or a spirit to them. They are animate and alive. Everything has a distinctive spiritual quality.

Throughout the continents, there was a similar sensitivity to who animals were. In Africa, people's daily needs have always been seen as associated with natural phenomena. In Asia, Jainism, Buddhism, Sikhism, Confucianism, Taoism, and Shinto share the concepts of dharma, karma, and reincarnation. The First People of Australia were nomadic people who came from southeast Asia. While they were hunters, they were very aware of the fragile nature of the earth. Aborigines believe that animal, plant, and human ancestors created the world and everything in it. They call this dreamtime.

In North America, Native American cultures viewed animals as equals in terms of rights. While they hunted, it was strictly for food. There was a connection made with the spirit of the animal and the hunting took place within a perceived permission. In Mesoamerican cultures of Central America, and reaching down to South America, the pre-Columbian era, some Mesoamerican cultures—Olmec, Aztecs, Maya, and Incas—did own livestock. They were more hunter-gatherer-based and had a deep reverence for the land and the animals. They held rituals that involved theatrical impersonation of situations and some of the ritual was represented by animals.

Before much of colonization, and subsequent missionary work, many tribes and cultures would subscribe to the same animism principles. The sighting of a certain animal may foretell or have significance for an event in the future. There was a deep reverence for, and connection to, the natural world and animals. As things have evolved, this has changed, largely due to the human/wildlife conflict. There is a revitalization around how important animals are to the culture of many formerly colonized places on Earth.

Here's the great news about Antarctica, no humans have screwed this up. Antarctica was part of a greater landmass . . . way before humans showed up in Africa. They exist in their own *umwelt*—an environment of their own.

Europe, and the part of Asia now considered the Middle East, had a different take on everything. Again, going back to the first chapter where I talk about "agriculture being born" in the Steppes area—ranging from China to Central Europe—we saw domestication and the working relationships between animals and humans begin.

From Aristotle to the dawn of the main religions we have today, the areas of Europe and the Middle East were the birthplace for speciesism. Speciesism is the practice of favoring one species over another—mainly humans over all else—which ultimately leads to the mistreatment and exploitation of animals.

The voice of the animal has been exponentially quashed, from trophy hunting, to poaching to food to drug testing, and even slips into the training mechanisms of the domesticated "friend" in our home.

As we discover their voice more and more and how much our dominance has led us to present day, we also see an increase in the many who are trying to improve how we listen to the voice of animals.

Fifth Chakra Emotions and Energetics

How often does our story, our expression about animals to others affect their ability to express who they are in life? Everything we say about them either lifts them up or gets stored in an energetic vault of entrapment that they are privy to. Labeling them as naughty, or the rescue, can keep them trapped in their title. Is there a gain to the story?

A young woman named Heidi had me come out to the barn where she boarded Jigs, her horse of several years. Jigs is a beautiful, gentle thoroughbred. When I got to the barn, I came into the stall, where Jigs stood elegantly eating. It was hard to imagine that there would be any challenge to their relationship as she seemed so acquiescent, with a nurturing quality.

I brought out my pen and paper and told Heidi what I tell everyone as I'm about to start the communication process, "I'm going to get quiet now and connect with your horse." No sooner had I settled into this quiet world when Heidi said, "Um, I should probably tell you that at the track, Jigs . . ." "Okay, thank you," I replied, and closed my eyes again.

"Oh and, Jigs . . ."

I smiled and nodded and acknowledged her comment. Again, upon silencing my mind, Heidi had to tell me one more thing about Jigs, and tell me about one more clinic she went to in order to fix the problems, or one more horse whisperer's observation about the horse. Perhaps, after this comment, Heidi realized that I might want to have quiet time, so she stopped.

Each of these stories were epic stories. Each of these stories were by rote, meaning, they were tried and true, she'd been sharing these stories about Jigs to anyone who would listen.

They were all things that could create confusion and/or mixed messages and were not easily remedied. However, I stayed with my connection with Jigs. Jigs confirmed these stories were true, yet that was not what was bothering Jigs.

In the world according to Jigs, Heidi had stopped praying or meditating, I couldn't tell which it was.

After the initial communication, I sat breathing and quieting myself again to find the best way to deliver the message. Finally, I asked Heidi how long she had been married. She told me six months. I said, "How would you feel if you went to dinner with your husband to meet some of his friends who you had never met. When you get in the restaurant lobby, your husband introduces you and says, 'This is Heidi, she had an abusive upbringing, just terrible. After that she drank too much in college and was a little wild for a while. She stopped that and is much better, and I think she'll behave tonight'?"

Heidi just stared at me for a moment.

As funny as that sounds, the truth is that we all do it to our animals. We bring the story into the lobby before the animal can arrive. We don't introduce our friends with, "Remember she's the one I was telling you about whose husband had an affair for six years?" Nor do we look at someone who is physically challenged and upon meeting them say, "God, what happened to you?" We also don't introduce people and say, "She's the one whose parents died in a fiery car crash when she was two, and she was passed from home to home."

Between humans, we demonstrate some manners, some decorum, some decency. There, see? We're not so bad! We observe, and perhaps comment on that. We allow the slow reveal, the information to trickle forth as the relationship deepens. We don't drag each other's stories around and watch it go from snowball to abominable snowman. Yet we have no problem doing this to and for our animals. We tell all in front of our animals. Nothing and nowhere is sacred—the dog park, in line at the feedstore. All of our friends know and even the guy at the grocery store knows a big secret about your challenges.

Getting back to Heidi . . . she was pretty stunned when I said this to her, yet she knew that this information was important. Additionally, the revelation her horse had about her prayer/meditation rituals was great for her to hear—even though she felt her horse had told on her—as she had slacked off, and felt guilty about that. Heidi enjoys a rich Christian life and truly incorporates prayer into her life. The horse could feel that Heidi was not actively grounding, and not being true to herself. So, in the end, the relationship shifted to a new level of peace and growth, and not for any of the reasons that Heidi was broadcasting.

Fifth Chakra Behavior, Dynamics, and Relationships

I was with Gabrielle for nearly 33 of her 36 years. She was an Arabian and Aries which meant, 100 percent fire. I met Gabrielle because she let out a high-pitched squeal to me as I was walking up the barn aisle to see my beloved horse, Pet One. The first time I thought to myself, I don't know this horse. I thought that up until that moment, Pet One was the most beautiful horse in the world, especially at the barn where I was boarding her. Now, here was a stunning mare, another beauty in the barn.

After that, every morning it became a routine. This stunning mare said hello in her lively horse talk, and I said hello to her in my human voice. I kept my eye out to see which person she belonged to. Then I discovered one Saturday morning, she belonged to a very cute guy, Tom. And we fell in love. We rode our two horses together into the sunset. For a brief time. But in that short time together, Pet One and Gabrielle bonded. We had lots of trail rides in Griffith Park, and our lives centered around our horses.

Even while we were together, Tom was very busy with work. He was a lawyer trying to become a partner in the big fancy firm he was working for. I found myself caring for Gabrielle because I was there every day anyway taking care of Pet One. At one point, Tom had sent Gabrielle off to a cowboy trainer. Gabrielle was never quite the same.

Even after Tom and I broke up, I couldn't not care for her, especially because he got so busy, nobody was taking care of her.

If you've read my first book, *Communication with all Life, Revelations of an Animal Communicator* (Hay House, 2007) then you will know that I tragically lost Pet One the night that she gave birth to Pony Boy. Tom eventually gave me Gabrielle.

Gabrielle was outspoken from the start, and she would swing her long mane around for dramatic emphasis. In many ways, that first whinny was her way of picking me, but it would take me many years to figure that out.

Once she was mine, our beginning was rough. I was in deep grief after the loss of my soulmate horse Pet One, and a bit in shock at having an orphan colt, Pony Boy. After being with the cowboy trainer, Gabrielle was very anxious. She would anticipate my every move, and it became quite frustrating—for both of us. Then we had a terrible accident in the Los Angeles River. I had a broken ankle, torn ligaments, and tendons. She was very sore on her front leg. We had matching leg wraps, only mine was a cast, and my ankle was held in place with a metal plate and five screws.

Once I recovered, Gabrielle and I still had some trepidation around certain things. She also had some soft tissue damage that would rear its mysterious head at times that I would least expect, and which always led me to question whether it was physical or behavioral.

In some ways we got further and further apart when it came to riding. Between having an orphan colt, Pony Boy, and a horse who didn't want to do dressage, I learned a ton of groundwork. And in that way, we truly connected. I loved dressage and found ways to ride other people's upper-level horses.

Eventually I got married and moved to Denver, where my husband was living. I added Rollie, my new dressage horse, to the mix. He loved to do what I did. At the same time, I tirelessly tried to find things to do with Gabrielle. We tried different trainers, different methods but always came back to groundwork.

In about the year 2000, after the fifteen-millionth tête à tête, we were walking back from another unsatisfying situation in the round pen—more groundwork—when I heard as loud as someone speaking directly to me, "It's hard to take direction from you, I've been your mother in so many lifetimes."

Well. There it was. And that changed everything. At least the fight.

We all moved to Florida, only to go through the same thing, try to find that thing she loved to do. We were always in barns where there was much activity, so it seemed like certainly there would be something we could do. Oh yeah, groundwork.

When I got divorced, my mom had been dead for a short time, and my dad was still alive. I moved back to the Seattle area—where I'm from—to help my family. My dream of living with my horses came true. I tried more with her and eventually just decided, she hated to be ridden. So that was that. Her only job was to be a horse. We walked through the woods together.

A few years after my dad died, we returned to California because both she and I craved sunshine. We had Anya in tow, and she continued to be a horse.

The relationship I had with her was like no other. The dynamic at times was contentious. Her favorite game was "I'm right and Joan's a dumbass." I have some of the funniest telepathic stories to prove how many times she won. I'm a Leo, she's an Aries, it could be big. Yet, I did more for that horse than any other being in my life. I moved several times so that she wouldn't be the odd man out. I moved onto horse property, so that she didn't have to be the only one not doing a "job." I created a herd. She got me to try every supplement there ever was and I learned more about nutrition and horses because of her. She shaped who I am today. In fact, it was her mystery lameness that got me to take a year-long animal communication course to get to the bottom of our issues. I learned TTouch to help her, acupressure, and myofascial release—all in the 90s. Eventually I added cranial sacral to the list. In California, I built a paddock paradise on my small piece of land so that she had to move all day on the track from water to food to water again—this replicates life in the wild. I even adopted a horse from a rescue to be her companion.

I learned to listen to her true essence, which was to be my best friend, my barometer, my touchstone, my equine better self. I loved caring for her until her very last breath. And we miss her every day.

Gabrielle was a fierce force for good with a tall agenda who masqueraded as a beauty queen with a distinct little nicker. That first neigh roped me in and helped me give voice to hundreds of thousands of animals.

Fifth Chakra Organs, Structure, and Meridians

Organs and Systems

The fifth chakra is blue. It is associated with the throat, thyroid, teeth, gums, parathyroid, trachea, hypothalamus, esophagus, and the vertebrae of the neck. It does not relate to a major organ; instead, it is exposed. Cerebellum, brain stem, and the lizard brain. The lizard brain is responsible for our drive for food and sex and our freeze, fight, or flight.

- Physiological systems at work here—Lymphatic system, which feeds and cleans vessels, organs, and helps the immune system.
- Endocrine systems at work here—Thyroid, parathyroid.
- Nerve plexus—Cervical plexus, a very complex neurological superhighway flowing to and from head and neck.
- Spine—Cervical, C1-C8.

Meridians

Governing Vessel (GV), Conception Vessel (CV), Liver (Li), Stomach (ST), Small Intestine (SI), Kidney (KI), Triple Heater (TH), Gallbladder (GB).

All these glands are part of the endocrine system. In Chinese medicine the endocrine system is associated with the energy of the kidney, and the kidney meridian.

Because the throat needs enough space to swallow food or water and take in air, I call this a drive-through meridian space.

Putting It All Together: A Pain in the Neck

- Hypothyroidism in horses and dogs, and hyperthyroidism in cats. These conditions affect moods and result in all sorts of skin and hair disorders.

- Dogs who are exuberant—when that free, fun, joyful exuberance gets yanked on, this makes them more exuberant and they express an even greater need to be free, fun, and joyful. This then becomes a bad biofeedback loop. Dog: express, and human: yank, over and over. It makes for a misunderstood dog, who probably needs to see a chiropractor or a holistic veterinarian who can help the thyroid that has been knocked out of place and which is creating havoc on the whole system.
- Many animals suffer from jammed necks or severe tightness in this area, that goes largely undetected. Tension here can even lead to seizures. Jammed necks pushing into the cranial bones can cause some types of aggression. Jammed necks can also create a "whiplash," effect, which can result in thyroid issues
- E-Collars (electric collars) deliver a small "shock," and this lands right in the throat chakra. They are often used to quell barking, and also used as behavior modification tools through negative reinforcement. The long-term use can be damaging to the thyroid and the tissue around it.

While allergies may be connected to other chakras or other reasons, certainly two cases come to mind.

Stories

Thor

Edith had recently adopted a dog named Thor. Thor is mighty, despite his size. He was the pride and joy of his original owner, Patricia, until Patricia had her second baby. His behavior became unpredictable and Patricia had to isolate him for long periods of time. On top of it all, his allergies became overwhelming. His congestion and discomfort were hard to watch, and expensive. With a toddler and a newborn, Patricia had to make a decision that she would never want to make.

Thor ended up in another home as a foster with the hope of adoption but that went south quickly. Again, Thor was isolated from the family, and the allergies worsened.

When he finally came to Edith's home, where she has other dogs and a husband, Thor was able to slowly unwind. He could safely express himself. As he became more comfortable and part of a family, his allergies slowly but surely went away.

Anya

My own horse Anya is also a perfect example of the allergy connection to non-expression. Anya came from a fancy dressage barn and a very known trainer. She is a very sensitive horse, so the pressure of training was a lot for her. She became unpredictable and not easy to ride or understand. She became so overly sensitive to everything, materials, fly spray, stress. She even developed a goiter. Anya became like the princess and the pea. Her old person used to make sure that the holistic veterinarian had golden needles for acupuncture. Anya allegedly was isolated from other horses because it appeared that she didn't like other horses or dogs. She became demanding for attention in a way that seemed neurotic.

When she came to me, she was my dream dressage horse. I didn't put any pressure on her. In fact, I didn't ride her for the first few months that she was home. I let her be part of a herd. She had dogs and horses around her. She didn't have the pressure of that level of work, or a competitive setting. Occasionally the goiter or hives would appear over the years, and that was my cue to take the stress level down in the environment so that she could be the queen of hearts she was meant to be.

And now she is retired and hangs out in the herd, and everything is on her terms now. She hasn't had an allergic reaction for years.

Gracie

Gracie is a beautiful Shepherd cross who lives with her brother, an adopted brother, as well as her person, Denise. Gracie can bark. And when I mean bark, it is like she is casting out a stay-away zone with a seven-foot circumference. If you move, the loud proud sound machine starts back up again with intent.

Denise had fostered Gracie and her brother when they were puppies. Gracie was packed up and sent off to her forever home, and it didn't go well. Gracie was returned to Denise as the foster, and she then adopted her.

What happened in those two years? It's anyone's guess. Whatever happened, she was constantly told she was bad, she was too much, all of the things that we can think at times when we are in puppy management zone. It was as if this imprinted her, and her own true voice was lost.

Denise is a graduate of my school, CWALU, and has utilized its resources to work with Gracie in helping her to calm down through animal communication and EFT.

Fleetwood

Erica called for some animal communication and EFT with her beloved Fleetwood, the horse of her dreams. Fleetwood is a noble fellow, loyal, and thoughtful. He came with a little baggage, as there had been high hopes placed on him from the original owner, followed by Fleetwood seeming to be a disappointment. So much of Erica's relationship with him has been unraveling his shutdown while stepping into her own true self.

Fleetwood had a fear of loud sounds, like a tractor in the barn aisle (which was daily) and didn't trust big trucks.

"I know where it came from, he was nearly hit by a big truck with his old owner. The person they were with shared that as they were about to go through the horse crosswalk, where they had the right of way, and a big truck sped up instead of slowing down. It was a very scary experience."

When I communicated with Fleetwood, another part of the experience revealed itself. As the truck was approaching, he could feel his old owner's fear and, being the noble fellow, he couldn't do anything about it. Then as the truck passed, he felt her outburst of anger.

As you can imagine, if you are the helpful-type steed, and you survived potential doom with a sense of being out of control, the ensuing angry burst from your owner really is the icing on the cake. In fact, the whole experience was like a little dome over him that never left, especially every time he encountered the revving engine sound, and the bigger vehicles coming closer. It turns out that the former owner had quite a temper, so Erica confirmed that this would definitely be part of the equation.

We did EFT Tapping on him for the panic and helplessness of the oncoming vehicle, and then we tapped on him about Fleetwood's feeling of quicksand that her anger seemed to expose.

After that tapping session, I hadn't heard from Erica, and I checked in to see if we needed to do more. She said: "No, it was a miracle!"

There is something that both Fleetwood and Gracie share that is very common with animals from rescues, shelters, and even horses who have been with a number of owners. These sensitive souls feel deeply. Whatever disappointment, anger, sadness, or even berating that humans do, it is imprinted onto them. When things are calm, they are fine but the minute the fight or flight comes in, or something changes, those old feelings wash over them like a sea foam that sticks.

These old stories, these old words, these old feelings have created not just a well-trodden neuropathway but a full-on six-lane highway to flight, fight, or freeze. Until these stories are released through animal communication, energy healing (EFT in particular), and bodywork, these animals revert to their flight, fight, or freeze.

The need for finding their true expression—whether that is the form of play, activity, relationships, and letting their story be heard through animal communication—is imperative with these sensitive souls.

Henry

One of the funny things that happened when writing my first book was that the editor, Angela, let me know that a few days after I delivered part of the manuscript to her, she tried an exercise from the book. She said that she allowed her dog Henry into her space, and she heard very loudly, "I'm not a little boy, I'm a man." She had to look around the room, even though she knew she was the only human in the space.

She was stunned. Here she is an editor on every metaphysical topic, one more famous than the next, but never did she expect that response from Henry . . . and, it gets better.

Henry had been a little naughty with her in terms of intimidation. He's a small white dog, yet he could snarl and snap at Angela! Once she acknowledged him being a man, and not a little boy, she realized that most of the time, she spoke in baby talk as if he was this little baby that would never grow up. Not only was he not a dog/baby, but he was also a man, and the man of the house.

Miraculously, his male dog/intimidation tactics backed off. He never growled or snapped again. He also had a little spring in his step as he would walk out the door, because his job, his purpose was known.

THE SIXTH CHAKRA—SEEING

"The third eye center is the place of your intuition and your ability to "see" the unseen, know the unknown, feel the intangible, and connect with the invisible world of Spirit. The third eye is the center for your higher intuition. Intuition is your ability to have direct access to the truth, independent of any type of logical or reasoning process."

—Margaret Ann Lembo, *Chakra Awakening: Transform Your Reality Using Crystals, Color, Aromatherapy and the Power of Positive Thought*

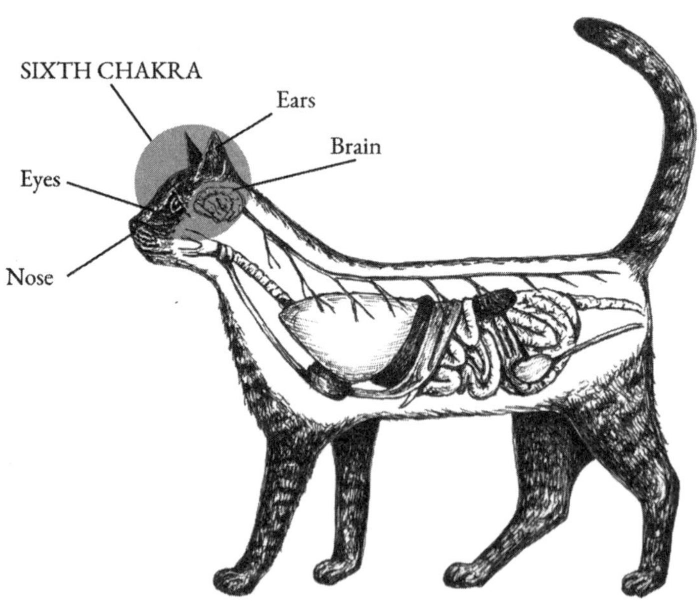

Fig. 7: The sixth chakra (third eye chakra)

Unicorns, Echolocation, and Sight Hounds—Oh MY!

If the eyes are the window to the soul, the third eye is window to all the dimensions. The third eye, the invisible eye, is known for the mystical and the unseen. We are going to go from the senses to intuition to the far-out and bring it all back again.

The physicality of the humans and animals we are primarily considering here has the eyes, ears, and sensory world right here in the third eye or the sixth chakra. While there are other beliefs around, the functions of the chakras and the senses, we are going to take a little leap here, and put the receptive fields (visual system, auditory system, and the somatosensory system) here.

In 1909, zoologist Jakob von Uexküll birthed the idea that the way that an animal perceives, senses, and experiences its surroundings is called *umwelt.* I can be typing this with my dogs and cats in the room and—while we are living in our shared ecosystem or morphic resonance (more on that in Chapter 8)—we are all experiencing this moment, and each other, from our own *umwelt.*

Science Journalist Ed Yong wrote an entire book around animals in their *umwelt* called *An Immense World, How Animal Senses Reveal the Hidden Realms Around Us* (Random House, 2022).

To me, in the same way that the fourth chakra brings together the worldly world and the unconditional love of the heart—and the universe for that matter—while connecting humans and animals, the sixth chakra brings together our ability to see things for what they are, our five senses, our sixth sense, and more. The sixth chakra shows the potential for seeing into other worlds, other dimensions, and others' realities. It gives us the capacity to understand beyond our 3D reality, and into the potential of string theory and ten-dimensional thinking, while also be the center of a sinus infection.

In other words, this space in our physical body is almost like a miner's hat with a beaming headlamp to understand and see into another being. We can detect and perceive our own experience here, as well as others'. And every being has this kaleidoscope experience as well, but in their own way with their own sensory abilities.

If we could truly see others, with detached compassion, and be neutral, this is the chakra where we could perceive our own animal's well-being and the multiverse all at the same time.

Ed Yong in *An Immense World* shares a hypothetical example to illustrate *umwelt.* He has the reader imagine a school gymnasium with an elephant, a mouse, a robin, an owl, a bat, a rattlesnake, a mosquito, a bumblebee, and a human all together. He then says that the robin can feel the season change coming up and that the earth's magnetic field guides the robin to want to fly south. He says:

"These seven creatures share the same physical space but experience it in wildly and wondrously different ways. The same is true for the billions of other animal species on the planet and the countless individuals within those species. Earth teems with sights and textures, sounds and vibrations, smells and tastes, electric and magnetic fields. But every animal can only tap into a small fraction of reality's fullness. Each is enclosed within its own unique sensory bubble, perceiving but a tiny sliver of an immense world."

As humans, we are very visually dominant. Our focus is on what we are perceiving through our sight. While many animals have good vision—the peregrine falcon's sight is better than ours—we rely largely on our sight, while maybe taking in the smells or sounds around us. Animals have a whole different experience. Being able to understand how their perception is shaped helps us to understand them better.

Eyes

Maybe we aren't going to solve global peace today, but we could end up understanding from the perspective of a horse that has their eyes on both sides of their head. I remember being in 4-H at school and having to do a Demonstration on sight. A 4-H Demonstration consisted of essentially picking a subject and creating a presentation about it. I was in 4-H and Pony Club for many years, but I went to state competition with my 4-H Demonstrations. My Demonstrations ranged from bones of the foot to lameness, to legs to eyeballs. This included how the horse eye worked. I made giant diagrams showing the wide field. My mom did the illustrations, my stick figures are imbalanced and ugly. Anyway, I couldn't believe how they saw. I must have been 12, but I never forgot. I don't know if I necessarily processed it well until later in life.

Indeed, that is part of the challenge of understanding another. Their perception is SO DIFFERENT to ours. The idea that the horse can see this giant field of vision to the side—and I look straight ahead—is truly mind boggling.

For a moment:

Imagine that you can't see something straight in front of you—about 6 inches wide—or directly behind you—just about the width of your tail—but somehow your eyeballs are capturing everything from each side all the way to your butt. Basically 340 degrees, and processing all of it. What's more, as a prey animal, you must decide if that thing that moved twenty feet away is after you. Okay, it was just a bird. Phew.

Most prey animals have eyes on each side of their head to have a better field of perception.

Most predators have forward-facing eyes. This helps with focus and depth perception to go after their prey.

Back to horses, the prey animal some of us have in our family. Apart from side vision, horses have dichromatic vision (colour blindness) as well. Their vision is much more complex. Imagine that they see basically to the side from both eyes, really each eye—ranging nearly three-quarters around behind them, leaving their behind very vulnerable. Not only that, but directly in front of them—a ways out—is a second blind spot.

When I think of how delicate the horse system is, I am mind blown daily that they allow us to be friends with them. It is one of the biggest honors of my life to feed and care for my horses daily. And I love to feel into their sight just for a moment each day.

There is a little difference in the sight of different dog breeds. The dogs bred for guarding and patrolling allegedly have nearsightedness (myopia) and the dogs bred for retrieving, and the sighthounds, are more farsighted (hyperopic). They say that dogs with flatter faces and shorter noses have sight similar to that of humans. (Which is funny how humanized little smush-faced dogs have become.) Again, dogs have the dichromatic vision, based out of two of the three color spectrums. They also have the *tapetum lucidum*, a layer of tissue that behind the retina, reflects light back through the retina.

Cats can see in low lights. They have very sensitive vision. Like dogs, they have the *tapetum lucidum*, as well as dichromatic vision.

Some birds, bats, toothed whales, and dolphins have something even cooler than sight. Their third eye has a melon-shaped receiver. They echolocate. That means, the melon-shaped sonar in their head can emit calls and listen to the echoes back of the object or being. Birds and bats use it for navigation, as well as foraging. Whales and dolphins in murky waters can see without seeing. They can find safety, as well as detecting predator or prey.

They can see without seeing, communicate without language, and be in that state of instinct and knowing all at the same time.

Imagine if we pretended to have a melon in our third eye and used it to echolocate our keys when they're lost—we'd probably do it faster than if we think it through logically. Imagine if we asked all of our senses to work together in unison all the time!

Ears

For horses, their hearing includes distinguishing between loudness, pitch, and localization, according to Janet L. Jones, Ph.D., in *Horse Brain, Human Brain, the Neuroscience of Horsemanship* (Trafalgar Square, 2020). This goes for many other animals who fall into the "prey" category.

Some interesting horse hearing facts:

- They hear us at lower volumes—what sounds to us as medium-loud will be very loud to a horse.
- They appear to listen to or react to things we can't hear.
- They are similar in octave range when it comes to pitch, but we hear lower frequencies and they can hear higher frequencies, things we can't hear like a high-pitched dog whistle.
- Horses are in for the win for localization. Their cupped ears help them to create a little Hollywood Bowl, and they can move up to 180 degrees backward and side to side. They can detect sound location in less than a degree of error—16 muscles make that happen as quick as a flick.

In her awesome book, she talks about interpreting sound, patterns of sound, and even music. But Janet shares a cautionary detail that many of us with sensitive horses know all too well:

> "Environments marked by loud, unexpected, and unfamiliar noises cause horses much distress. Even consistent unpleasant noises bother horses, like wind or idling diesel engines. Wind makes things flap around and engines mask sounds that might be important to a prey animal. Decades of research prove that constant noise is not good for human ears, minds, or emotions either. Animals—and humans—cannot relax in such settings, and without the security of relaxation, true learning is impaired."

A dog's hearing far surpasses the human auditory spectrum and frequently they can detect the exact location of a sound.

Here's why:

- Dogs have a deeper ear canal to funnel to the ear drum.
- They have 18 muscles in the ear flap (pinna) to move the ears to aim at and locate a specific sound.
- Once the sound enters the ear canal, it is amplified in the drum and the tiny bones.
- They have larger ears, and we can all hear the sly wolf telling Little Red Riding Hood that it is "all the better to hear you with, my dear."

According to Joshua Leeds and Susan Wagner in *Through a Dog's Ear: Using Sound to Improve the Health and Behavior of your Canine Companion* (Sounds True, 2008):

> "Over-stimulation leads to sensory confusion, due to the inability either to process input as fast as it is arriving or to put the input in context. We know that the impact of over-stimulation (i.e., chronic sound stress) on the human

> nervous system can be debilitating. What about an animal's nervous system? Does Lassie respond the same way you or your children do?"

I can't even tell you how many times I've communicated with dogs who were in the show ring or at an agility trial who completely lose their composure or the sense of what they are doing due to overstimulation of sound. Sometimes it is like the sound is up in the vast air of the stadium or building and then there is a gnawing buzz around them (of the people and dogs). The acoustics in these buildings are often not supportive of focus.

Cats' hearing is off the chart compared to human and they can perceive frequencies that are undetectable to humans. This they use for hunting primarily. They also can hear electricity! Like dogs, the sound rolls down the ear canal and amplifies in the eardrum. They also have quite a few muscles at work moving their ear around to be able to locate exactly where the sound is coming from.

Nose

Science focuses more on vision than any other sense. Vision and hearing are mechanical. When it comes to taste and smell, this produces chemistry. Smell for most animals, including human animals, is the very first part of the digestion process.

Horses love to put their soft nostril right on a human to get a sense of just who they are. It is like reading braille for them. A stallion can detect a mare from a mile away. Horses can understand with a few sniffs in the air where water is, where predators are, where other horses are, recognize another (animal or human) from long ago, and find their way home.

A dog's nose really does have superpowers. Their nostrils have superpowers. We've been hearing more and more about their need to sniff and the power of their nose. Because of their shape and the muscles lining the inside, they can sniff a smell, be exhaling but still pulling that scent in deeply and allowing it to sit in the olfactory bulb. That's where they get the download of information. Each nostril can sniff independently and receives different information. There is the long sniff, this is directional, air-pulling, and investigative. For nearby sniffs, they scan the surface, as if they're "not finding the smell" but all the while they not only are "on it" they are discerning, measuring, discovering, comparing, contrasting, surmising, and revising, all at the same time.

Cat's may have an even better sense of smells than dogs. Except for a few breeds of dogs with extra scent receptors, cats actually have way more receptors. In fact, it is said that cats smell their meals, rather than taste food. Cats have an extra benefit in that not only do they smell for the usual things, but they also have a vomeronasal up in the roof of their mouth and it can detect pheromone signatures. They have scent glands on their forehead, chin, lips, and tail to mark their territory. They smell for socialization, mating, hunting, and exploring the world.

EXERCISE

Take some long breaths in and sit with the slow breathing. Now takes some sniffs. Pick up whatever is next to you and sniff it. Really take it in and ponder what you smell.

Touch/Tactile

Horses use their whiskers, which are big, long sensory hairs. These whiskers have their own nerve and blood supply. It is a tactile feedback loop on their environment and surroundings. The whiskers help to fill in the blind spot horses have right in front of them. They even help them judge the distance of things around them since they don't see down that direction—unless they cock their head with their eyes facing straight down.

A horse can feel a fly land on its back and twitch the skin to get rid of it. Yet they love mutual grooming—they can put some muscle behind it and appear forceful which, in turn, can erupt into a "playful discussion," before going back to soft teeth!

Horses love a good massage from their human or the human their human hired! If it is their own special person, this may not only be a feel-good experience for the horse, but it can also be very bonding. And, massage can drop the heart rate. So, this is very good for all those horses who go into fight or flight in a moment.

The hoof is made of the same material as fingernails. The surface has no feeling, yet, what is under the fingernail or hoof outer layer is so sensitive. It is very protective. That protective layer enables them to do long-distance travel. The horse feels itself when its hoof hits the ground. The nerve endings respond and message the brain, "Here is ground!" In other words, it is a grounding.

Dog whiskers are so sensitive that they can detect environmental change, spatial differences, and even temperature, and wind speed.

Cat whiskers can help cats right themselves midair during a fall. The ends of the whiskers have proprioceptors (sensory receptors) that can help cats navigate their surroundings, and land on their feet! The root of the whisker is full of nerve endings to help them detect and navigate. Cat whiskers communicate what is going on—what you see is what you get!

Dogs and cats share a tactile sense of pressure, pain, and temperature. Dogs will groom each other, and they can easily get into a habit of licking due to anxiety, or allergies. Generally, they love being groomed or stroked by us. Cats, on the other hand, need to groom themselves to stabilize temperature, to stimulate circulation, and to eliminate parasites, infections, and allergies.

While many cats like being stroked, many of us have been smacked by the paw when overstimulation kicks in around mid-back, on the third or fourth stroke. Their skin has a high-density nerve endings. Cats know how to groom each other without hitting that hiss point.

Dog paw pads are a little fatter to deal with temperature changes. The "fat" helps to create balance, traction, stability, and shock absorption. Cat paws have nerve endings, and glands, to help navigate balance, traction, and feeling vibration (of potential predators).

EXERCISE

"The foot feels the foot when it feels the ground." The foot hitting the ground sends so many messages about the world around us. Take a moment and breathe into the bottom of your feet. Just be here for several breaths. This is the start of many meditations for Communication with all Life University and my wildlife trips.

Vibration, Frequency, and Electromagnetic

The third eye is the epicenter of processing all of this information from a truly energetic, vibrational, frequency, electromagnetic, and physical integration.

Magnetoreception is a thing! We all have receptors to understand the magnetic field. Everyone from our four-leggeds to our whales, dolphins, and sea turtles have this navigation center. The electromagnetic receptors are amplified by the minerals in the ground.

Our domesticated animals sense the electromagnetic field and use it as a compass. Certainly, all wildlife depends on their ability to feel it.

It is believed that migrating birds and many other birds can actually see the earth's magnetic field. There are molecules—in their eyes or brains—that detect and respond to magnetism. Peter Hore of Oxford University says that the molecules in the bird's eyes are responding to cryptochromes—light-sensitive proteins found in plants and animals that are said to be related to the circadian clock (the internal rhythmic clock of all living things). Hore believes that dusk activates this magnetic sense.

Others argue that migratory birds are simply seeing magnetic patterns of north and south, and this is what they follow. Salamanders and frogs also use a magnetic sense for orientation.

More Unique Ways of Sensing and Seeing with Sound

Animals who are blind practically see out of this third eye. It is as if they see without seeing. I have spoken to the guardians of many dogs, cats, horses, and more who have expressed the sentiment: "It's like they can still see."

It may be all the senses at work. One could say that the third eye is sonar-like. So, the sensors create an ability to see/feel into the world. Take the prey animals, the sensation follows the same pattern that their vision does.

EXERCISE

Close your eyes for a moment and imagine that you are a prey animal. You could be a bunny, a horse, an antelope. For a moment, imagine your sight actually expands all the way to your hind end. Now imagine connecting the vision and all the senses, all the while sensing out into the world around—creating an energetic bubble of safety.

The scientific community is still trying to figure out in the case of bats as to whether their sonar is a coherent field, which would mean that the sending and receiving is more of a state or field. The alternative theory is that bat's sonar sound bounces off the object and is then sent back within a fraction of a second.

Toothed whales emit a beam out of their third eye. The beam is transformed into clicks that come out of a place in the brain referred to as the "melon," located (in the third eye) in the concave bone of the cranium. A mass of fatty tissue found in the foreheads of all toothed whales, the melon focuses and modulates the animal's vocalizations ("clicks") acting as a sound lens. Again, two senses— sound and sight— are combined in the third eye region. In echolocating, bottlenose dolphins and porpoises also emit "clicks."

Some nocturnal birds, as well as shrews and a few other mammals like bats, have this echolocation. This helps not just to figure out predator versus prey and safety, but also helps to navigate through trees and bushes in the dark.

- Toothed whales—orcas and sperm whales, for example—use the larynx to seal the airway and have a vocal organ in their nose that makes sounds.
- Some fish, snakes, and insects have a "pit" that "sees" in infrared and actually detects the heat of another.

Unicorns and Rhinos

What came first, the unicorn or the rhino? Turns out, they were alive at about the same time. The rhinoceros, our big tank of an animal with a horn, has been evolving for 50 million years. There are five species of rhino—Indian, Sumatran, Javan, black, and white.

The black and white rhinos, both living in Africa, are actually all grey—the difference is that one has wider lips than the other because of the foraging that they do:

- Black rhinos have a pointed upper lip, while white rhinos have a squared lip.
- Black rhinos browse on leaves from trees and bushes, while white rhinos graze on grass.

They have evolved to have terrible sight, but great smell and hearing. The word rhinoceros comes from the Greek—*rhis* for the nose, and *keras* for the horn. Rhinos are poached mercilessly for their horn. Sadly, there are only two northern white rhinos left in the world. I have met them both and spent time with them on one of my wildlife trips.

We will come back to that.

Unicorns were somewhere between a horse and a goat in size, with a magical horn. According to Diana Cooper in her book *The Wonder of Unicorns* (Findhorn Press, 2019):

> "They are great healers, who can help you think and feel differently. They touch your third eye and your heart with the incredible light. This raises your frequency above the mental and emotional sources of dis-ease."

Unicorns were part of the Indus Valley (what is now between Pakistan and India), Egypt, and Mesopotamia (what is now the Middle East). They became part of Greek mythology, and the Bible. In mythology, while unicorns were difficult to capture, to drink a cup of magic from the horn of a unicorn was to stop epilepsy, stomach disorders, and more.

In the Bible, they were referred to as *re'em*, which could have been wild auroch, rhinoceros, or unicorn. The stories are more allegorical. It turns out they are so fast, that the only way to stop a unicorn is to throw a virgin at it.

Whether Mesopotamia, Egypt, Indus Valley, or the Bible, there seemed to be something magical with that horn.

During our early evolutionary history, there was a Siberian unicorn who became extinct about 350,000 years ago. It was an ox-like animal with a horn, looking very much like a rhinoceros. They existed at the same time as rhinos in early history.

In art, the unicorn has been depicted throughout European, Islamic, and Asian cultures.

Sadly, this has become like a bad game of "telephone" where every time the story gets told, it changes its truth a bit. And somehow, the rhino horn is one of the hottest commodities in Asia and is believed to have medicinal powers.

Meanwhile, whether you believe in unicorns in the real, or more magical sense, the rhino horn is keratin, the same as a horse's hoof, or our fingernails, and has no more medicinal power than chewing your nails.

Despite that, rhinos are being killed for their horns every eight hours by poachers in South Africa. And in other parts of Africa, daily, maybe not at such a staggering rate. Still, the rate of poaching is off the charts. It is so heartbreaking.

All that aside, the magic of unicorn energy is like nothing else. I feel like I live with a unicorn, my new horse Pegasus, he came to me in the last year. I wish I had a unicorn horn, or an echolocation "melon," or an extra 12 million dollars!

Third Eye and Other Dimensions

Many people ask me why their animal is staring at the wall or barking at the corner. They believe that their animals are seeing ghosts, or spirits of some form. It is certainly more than possible that there are more dimensions than our 3D world of width, height, and depth—up and down, and left and right. While string theory (which is more than ten dimensions) has not been solidified by science, the unified field has remained a consistent theory. Scientists and physicists are in it for the long haul to prove other dimensions. They wouldn't be following this persistently for hundreds of years now if there wasn't some sort of possibility. And just because there aren't spatial dimensions, new places that our experience doesn't allow us to see, it doesn't mean it doesn't exist. I mean, isn't that the theory of Heaven?

And how do we know our animals don't experience it? They wouldn't question it or have a belief in it one way or another. It would just be.

Cats have been associated with paranormal activity. Halloween portrays cats as part of the mystery being to accompany the witch. Cats have been perceived as magical and mystical throughout history, dating back to Egypt.

The processing center behind the third eye is where all of the senses would measure a unified field from. And some animals seem to be moving through the world as if they are perceiving other dimensions all the time. We just have no alleged proof.

Yet, we see birds flying in a pattern using the earth's magnetic field for navigation.

The wavelengths in our own perception don't allow us to see the magnificent colors a mantis shrimp can see. Many animals have such a different eyeball structure or eye placement, so naturally they see differently than we do. Who's to say they are not seeing into another dimension? Certainly, their behavior and communication make it clear they are seeing something else.

Sixth Chakra Symbolism

The sixth chakra is where all of the senses come together and are perceived. The sixth chakra centre is responsible for cosmic perception (other dimensions included in that), energy flow, intuition, wisdom, and fulfilling desires. It acts as the intermediary between consciousness and an individual's inner world.

This center, especially when focused upon during meditation, is where seekers search for the answers, truth, the meaning of life, desires, and reality. While animals aren't necessarily questioning in this same way, they are being in their senses no matter how evolved we perceive them to be.

Sixth Chakra Species-Specific/Wild and Domestic

Two legs and a head is what I call an animal in fight or flight. Whether it is our own dog, cat, horse, or the gazelle on the fly. The adrenals shoot off, the lungs expand, the brain chemistry fires, and they are off. Their head gets higher (or in the case of cats, sometimes lower), and it's as if they forgot their hind end and the race is on with all the weight on the front end and, something, divine guidance is leading. The third eye is like a miner's hat with a light beaming straight ahead.

Many animals also have a *tapetum lucidum*, a layer on the back of the eye that acts like a mirror. That's why, when you flash a light on them, you can see the light reflecting back at you. It helps them to see better at night, and they look scarier to us!

The other supercool protection that many species have is the nictitating membrane—it's referred to as a third eyelid. This comes in handy if you are a dive-bombing peregrine falcon leaping off a mountain at 200 mph. If you are a polar bear, this protects you from becoming snow-blind. Many other reptiles and birds have this protection. It is there for dogs and cats but tucked high up and can only be seen when gently opening an animal's eye.

Animals in the wild are dependent upon their senses for survival. After years of research and studies of the social life of elephants, a field scientist, Caitlin O'Connell, discovered their communication through the ground; the seismic vibration of the earth allowed the elephants to listen through their limbs and respond or react accordingly. In her book *The Elephant's Secret Sense, The Hidden Life of the Wild Herds of Africa* (Chicago Press, 2007), she states:

> "For the elephants in the wild, I was beginning to think that seismic signals played an important role in their complex communication repertoire. Perhaps they, too, had honed their skills at detecting vibrations to better interpret their world."

Her research and development of this seismic theory led to a deep understanding and relationship with these elephant families. She was then able to work with the local governments in Namibia to deter the wild animals from raiding villager's crops and work toward a peaceful approach to cohabitation and promote conservation.

The Shadow Side of the Sixth Chakra

If you were to do a search on Google of electromagnetic fields and horses, you will see all the products that are available to help horses, with everything from magnetic leg wraps to vibration machines to help circulation. While all of these products are great (and I have plenty), they are geared toward the "performance" of the horse.

Rarely is it noted that the things that are hindering their performance, changing their behavior, creating restlessness, weird immune responses, and reactivity is that our invasion of electromagnetic disturbances has left them uneasy. They can feel the powerlines, an electric fence, appliances, bad lighting in barn aisles and arenas, transformers, Wi-Fi routers, and more.

Often there will be a "spooky corner" in an arena. I remember boarding my horses in Los Angeles and we called the public arena down the street the "spooky arena," which was not far off the I-5 freeway, and under some hefty powerlines.

Light Pollution

The glow of artificial lighting takes its toll on wildlife, domestic animals, and human's circadian rhythm. For songbirds migrating at night, it can completely disorient them and throw them off course. Millions of sea turtle hatchlings die because they move toward the light rather than the direction of the ocean. Some cities along Florida's east coast have taken measures to stop the city lights and have volunteers protecting these babies.

As much as we admire the city lit up in the distance, it wreaks havoc on natural systems. Europe is the most light-polluted continent.

Noise Pollution

Noise-induced hearing loss affects all of us. Machines, loud music, airplanes, you name it, we've all been susceptible to it. And so are our animals at home. But the ramifications are even worse for wildlife. Think of fireworks going off. What warning do our wild friends get, and where do they go?

What creates noise pollution? Propellers, ferries, cargo ships, and more. It becomes audio chaos. Noise pollution is at a critical point with marine life. Recent studies show that the noise in the ocean is affecting the fish and all invertebrates.

The Salish Sea is home to several pods of some of the most endangered orcas on the planet. When I did naturalist training ten years ago, the population was 93. Now it is 74. The biggest killer? Noise pollution.

Because the Salish Sea is one of the biggest shipping lanes for consumer goods coming in and out of the US, plus the oil pipeline from Canada, the vessel traffic from tankers has tripled. It hinders hunting because orcas see with sound. Their echolocation gets thrown off and creates an inability to find food.

"The noise is analogous to foggy conditions where the whales are unable to see as far using echolocation," Dimitri Ponirakis—a noise analyst at Cornell University, U.S., who wasn't involved in the study—told Mongabay in an email. "This means that they must expend more energy to find the same amount of prey as they would under normal ambient conditions."

Sixth Chakra Emotions and Energetics

Memory, guilt, thought, and ego are all considered part of the sixth chakra.

I always say there is no negative emotion for an animal, it is all about survival. Fear, panic, and even rage are all built to put an animal in fight or flight mode. It becomes their GPS system to get them up and out of the situation or to fiercely fight for what is theirs. In other words, for animals, these "negative" emotions are all built to save their lives. In my classes I regularly say there are no positive or negative emotions, simply emotions.

In her book *Horse Brain, Human Brain: The Neuroscience of Horsemanship*, Janet L. Jones explains:

> "Brain chemicals cause emotions to create especially strong memories. When an event occurs that triggers fear, for example, the brain releases stress hormones corticosterone, vasopressin, and epinephrine. These chemicals prepare the body for a fight or flight response and set the memory of that event in neural concrete. Why? Because to survive, we must remember fearful experiences—they're dangerous and need to be avoided in the future."

She goes on to say that learning should be done in the setting of tranquility, curiosity, and trust. And this is true for animals and humans.

Sixth Chakra Behavior, Dynamics, and Relationships

Charly is a very tall, handsome horse who is being leased by Joni. When Joni had me out to communicate with Charly, she told me that he spooked on the trails and that it was very scary. Joni wants to do cross country (which is jumping out in a field—and some trails) and this was not possible with his spookiness.

When I connected with Charly, he told me he was very smart, he loved to be in connection with Joni, he was very true, he loved to work, and all the things you'd want to hear from a horse that you were going to partner with in a sport.

When I did the animal medical intuition scan, I sensed that he heard differently in each ear, like one ear was slightly muffled. He detected high-pitched sounds, but he couldn't place where they were coming from. And I sensed his back would tighten and he would stick his head high in the air. Joni said that is exactly what happens. She said that even when walking him off the property, he has his head in the air.

When we did EFT (Emotional Freedom Technique) Tapping on him, I addressed the fact that he didn't know where sound was coming from and that he was scared. We ended with the desired outcome of "No matter where the sound was coming from, he was safe with Joni."

Joni and I then walked him off the property in the equestrian neighborhood where he lived. Every yard had a horse that was ready to say hello. But to our surprise, Charly wasn't interested. He had his nose to the ground smelling the world. Joni couldn't believe it, she said she had never seen him that relaxed. The tapping released his need to depend on his ears.

In the distance, a work van for a cable company was parked on the side of the road with a ladder going up into the trees (could be truly scary stuff for a horse). Then, as if on cue, a man came off the ladder (Charly was still smelling) and opened the back door of the van with the worst creaky sound you've ever heard. Like nails on a chalkboard creak. Charly's head shot up and he froze, his ears pointing every direction.

I said, "Joni, tell him where the sound is coming from."

Joni said, "Charly, the horrible sound came from that van over there." Joni pointed to the van. His eye followed the movement of her hand and his sight settled on the van for a moment. None of the other horses in the neighborhood reacted.

And within a beat, Charly went back to sniffing the road. He has been great on the trail since—and he uses all of his senses now.

Sixth Chakra Organs, Structure, and Meridians

Organs

The sixth chakra can be purple, violet, indigo, or white. It governs the pineal and pituitary glands, the brain, eyes, ears, nose, cerebrum, amygdala, and hippocampus.

The amygdala is the emotional thermostat. It is in charge of fear and all of the deep visceral emotions. It is part of the limbic system, a neural network, and is involved with emotion and memory. It is a group of nuclei, or clusters of neurons.

The hippocampus is similar to the amygdala in that it is a paired structure. It is responsible for holding memory, particularly long-term memory. It is also needed for spatial understanding and navigation.

Humans have a prefrontal cortex in this sixth chakra, third eye area. Dogs and cats have a very small prefrontal cortex. Horses have none. The prefrontal cortex is responsible for organizational thinking, planning, goal setting, executive thinking.

- Physiological systems at work here: Endocrine (while it works in every chakra, this is communication central), and limbic system.
- Endocrine systems at work here: Pineal gland, and pituitary gland.
- Limbic systems at work here: Amygdala, and hypothalamus.

- Brain area: Prefrontal cortex.
- Nerve plexus: Cranial nerves (12 nerves in the back of the brain responsible for face, neck, torso, and sensations).
- Spine/Skeleton: The axis, atlas, occipital, and sphenoid bones, temporal, mandible, and many of the facial bones.

The Vagus Nerve travels through:

- Lungs
- Spleen
- Liver
- Kidney
- Small Intestine
- Colon
- Brain

Meridians and Traditional Chinese Medicine

Governing Vessel (GV), Small Intestine (SI), Triple Heater (TH), Gall-bladder (GB).

- The stomach meridian (yang) starts under the eye, comes down to the mouth, travels up to the ear and then back down on the belly, ending on the inside of the back legs.
- The heart (yin) meets up with the spleen meridian in the armpit and follows down the inside of the front legs.
- The small intestine (yang), on the other side of the foot from the heart meridian, follows up the outside of the front leg, up the shoulder, and up the temporomandibular joint to the ear.

Putting It All Together: It's All About the Head

- blindness
- eye disorders
- ear disorders
- headaches
- neurological disorders
- learning disabilities
- tumors
- strokes
- seizures
- sinus challenges (often referred to as uncried tears)
- memory issues
- vestibular disease

Head injuries cause so many of the conditions listed above. But they also change the personality, and sometimes the trajectory, of the animal. Sometimes animals get to a point of never quite perceiving things in the same forward-thinking way that they used to. Because we can't necessarily see their pain or know exactly what happened—they may have jammed their neck jumping off the bed, or T-boned another dog at the dog park while you turned away that one second—suddenly you have either a mystery behavior, or a seizure.

Dolphins, the Super Facilitators

My friend, James Nemec, was a wonderful craniosacral bodyworker, as well as a great writer. He spent many years working with the Upledger Institute in the Bahamas, where they would do craniosacral work in the water and the wild dolphins were free to come in and participate in the healing or go about their business. He called the dolphins super facilitators. In his book *Touch The Ocean: The Power Of Collective Emotions* (CraniOcean Media, 2007), he says:

> "What I mean by super facilitators is that dolphins, like the very best body workers and massage therapists, meet you where you are. They have no judgment on who or what you ought to be. They meet you where you are without regard to nationality, religion, race, creed, smell. This is a lesson in itself. Each dolphin responds precisely to where you are, moment by precious moment, in thought and in feeling."

He goes on to say that there is an invisible boundary and that while it feels personal on the one hand to be met at that level, on the other hand it is intimate while being impersonal.

When I was in the naturalist program there, there were all of these stories . . . of orcas sensing pregnancy, the vibration of the active womb would draw the orcas to the pregnant woman.

Stories

My Own Sister Is Living Proof: The Dolphin Story

Growing up, I was the oldest of two sisters, and a brother. My sister, Laurie died in 1986 of a brain tumor. It could be said that it started my whole journey into alternative health, healing, and ultimately animal communication. A few years later, my other sister, Mary, was diagnosed with a life-threatening disease. It was not looking good. In fact, I was still in therapy, working through my grief about Laurie, and was starting to do the work of the potential loss of Mary. Spoiler alert, Mary is still alive. I attribute this story as to why.

My mother's answer to facing any kind of grief or hardship was to book a trip somewhere. Especially if someone had some last wishes. Mary wanted to swim with dolphins. My mother suggested we go to

South Florida—Miami, Key West, and Key Largo—where we could swim with dolphins.

It was 1989 we were set to go to the Dolphin Research Center in Key Largo. The dolphins allegedly are free to come and go. I'm not so sure about any of that but when you know better, you do better. I would never swim with dolphins in captivity again but, this is about my sister.

When I met my mom and Mary in Miami, I hadn't seen her for a couple of months. While we talked regularly, I wasn't prepared for how bloated Mary was from the medication, her face was puffed up, she had marshmallows for cheeks. Her fair, freckled skin was opaque except for the makeup that was unevenly dabbed on. Her hair looked like straw, and she wore dark glasses to protect her overly sensitive eyes. My mother would toss a glare across to me as if to say, "I told you she was bad."

Getting the rental car took forever. The ease of conversation we had had on the phone was muted by my shock. My mom was dealing with her own health issues so the weight that Mary had gained wasn't on our side as we got her in and out of the wheelchair. My heart sank. I didn't know how I was going to manage a week with now my second sister in a rapid decline. How was my mom assisting a second daughter to her death? What was my mother thinking, bringing what was basically a shell of my sister, a breathing blob on a trip? And how did she talk me into this?

After much struggle amongst what to wear, getting Mary in and out of the rental car, wheelchair, the new and not improved dull Mary due to the drugs, we finally arrived at the dolphin research center the next morning. There was only one other girl signed up with us. We had the whole place to ourselves.

After the customary safety guidelines, we helped Mary into the pool. I got in, as did the other gal that was in our time slot. On demand, the dolphins came tumbling in to greet us. I was so excited; I didn't expect the moment of overwhelm I had at this large swimming being with such a big intention. It's easy to misread that anatomical smile on the dolphin, but in this moment, I took it as real. And in no time after sliding around and being in their presence, even if it was in captivity, the pool water was infused with glee.

Was it mine? Was it Mary's? Was it the other girl? Was it from the dolphins? Did somebody purposely inject glee into the pool chemicals each night when they checked the pH? No matter, it was bubbling up and infectious.

Because there were only three of us and maybe we had bad dolphin trainers, it was somewhat of a free for all. I remember the sense of the dolphins paying equal attention to us and being very curious. The trainers were prepared to show us all the "tricks" they do, including hanging on to the dorsal fin and going for a ride. None of us cared to do that. We were quite happy being with them.

Later, we had lunch there and did a tour. Again, the place was completely empty. So, my mom organized a second swim. We spent the afternoon with dolphins, a lazy trainer, and moved through time and space with two dolphins who were assigned to swim with us. The trainer knew we didn't have those expectations of tricks and such so we spent time dipping under and over dolphins. Heaven.

When we got to Key West, we were exhausted and checked into our hotel. The next morning, I rose before anyone did. When I travel—unless on safari with lions outside—I get up and take a walk after I meditate. As I was trying to sneak out before the light came up, Mary asked me where I was going.

"On a walk, and then to get coffee." Mary never liked coffee. Between her illness and the end goal of a latte, I was surprised to hear, "Wait for me."

The rented wheelchair remained in the trunk of the rental car. Each day we woke up and had some sort of aquatic adventure, snorkeling, boat rides, lunch out on another island, even jet skis. Mary was suddenly the adventurous little sister I had always known.

I have to say, I know it was the dolphins. They had a sense from her and beamed something to her. And my mother knew exactly what she was doing. As always.

My Echolocation Experiments

The idea that we could potentially tap into this third eye like echolocation had me intrigued for a while, to say the least, so I decided to try it out:

I was living outside of Seattle at the time in a town called Carnation. I was on 23 acres, with an open pasture but surrounded by woods. When it was dark, it was dark. Each stall had a run (a small paddock) off of it. And my horse Rollie—a tall, dark thoroughbred—loved to stand guard in his paddock. He was a ladies' man after all, and he had to protect my other two horses, Gabrielle, and Anya. Rollie wouldn't rush in like the others to get that late night mash and more hay.

I would walk into his stall and close my eyes and stand in the doorway to the run. I would determine where the big object (Rollie) was. I was feeling with my third eye if I could sense where the center of this heartbeat was, the blood coursing through veins with a charming electromagnetic field. Then I would walk toward this thing.

Many times, I would reach Rollie's rib cage and touch him as if I found the piñata. But a few times I ended up at the fence and would open my eyes only to look over at Rollie across the paddock. He would throw a quick look that could only say, "You dumbass, I'm over here."

And my favorite was when a bat flew into me in the third eye. Rollie loved our third eye games and didn't come into the stall for his late-night tuck-in until I had completed my assignment.

Maggie

When I arrived, Maggie, a picture-perfect black lab was sitting in the back of the truck bed, overlooking a park-like yard that had views for miles of the Olympic mountains on this particular gorgeous Seattle morning. She appeared serene and settled in her ritual of taking in the morning smells and bird calls.

At the time of my visit to meet Maggie she was ten, yet she seemed ageless. She had been blind since she was six. Audra, her lovely human, had said her sight had been gradually diminished due to a degenerative disease but that now there was something even worse happening with the eyes. Audra had me come out to discuss the upcoming surgery, during which her eyes would be removed.

When I communicated with Maggie, she said she was okay with the upcoming surgery. One of the reasons Maggie was okay with it was because of Sam, she said.

Sam was their other dog. Audra and her husband had adopted Sam when Maggie was about five. Sam had a troubled start and was a little bit difficult to settle at first, and then something miraculous happened. Sam became Maggie's eyes.

Audra said that the way the two dogs moved through the trails together, you would never know Maggie was blind. Many people were surprised to find out she was blind. Audra also shared she would often see Maggie move through the house as if she still had her sight.

Gremlins

Petunia is the dog of a skilled energy clearing expert, Nancy. Nancy and Petunia had recently lost the other dog in the household and were both grieving. When Nancy made the appointment, she had said that Petunia was much more anxious. When I checked in with Petunia, she shared that Nancy wasn't herself. That Nancy had done a big clearing, but stuff hadn't left. Petunia said she could still see the gremlins and she was worried when Nancy would walk out the door into the world. It was this image of almost wanting to hand Nancy an umbrella or pack her lunch!

Nancy shared that she had a clearing on herself by another professional and it felt more like an exorcism! She said that there was residual energy in the house. By acknowledging that Petunia could see all of the energy that Nancy was working with, we were elevating Petunia in the household. And Nancy knew that as the emotional leader of the household she had to convey more confidence.

Watching the Senses at Work

That same horse Rollie had a thing for my little cat, Queen Latifah. While she is more petite, she makes up for it in personality size. Yet, she would suddenly seem demure when she came to his stall, and ask to be picked up, and carried like a baby. He would put his left nostril on her side and gently inhale and exhale three times. Her eye would soften, and the little ritual was complete. This played out a few times a week for years. I figured they had some sort of past life relationship and by bringing them together, I was facilitating their reunion.

Sensing and Seeing Coyotes on Our Dog Walks

Since I've been working on this chapter, I've been hyper aware of my own animal senses and what I've witnessed in the wild. It has been enlightening!

On so many safaris, I've seen the senses be the only thing between life and death for prey animals. On a trip to Hwange National Park in Zimbabwe, we were parked next to a pride of juvenile lions basking in the sun, in a pile like housecats. There were four girls and one boy. The boy was out, like he could sleep in like a teenager. The girls had eyes shut but nostrils at work. And ears.

They blended into the scenery. Off in the distance, the watering hole was a perfect target for any potential hunt. We watched as a single zebra would show up to drink, with a herd in the distance. The pride would be captivated (except for our dear boy) and ears up, eyes open, all from a scent.

The light breeze would redirect and suddenly, without sight or hearing, the zebra was aware and galloping off with the distant herd in tow.

That fast. Just off of a scent.

My dogs and I hike out into the hills of Santa Clarita several mornings a week. Coyotes blend into the golden hills in the same way lions do in the African bush. My Penelope has some sight hound in her and can see something and then Abby, my lab/shar-pei will get those nostrils working and then my eyes catch sight of the coyote ears popping out of the tall dry grass. My dog, Delilah sometimes sees and sometimes smells. But it is game on. And thankfully, they are relatively well trained, and we leave the coyotes alone. But we bark!!

It has brought an appreciation and awareness as to what we lead with. While humans are very visually driven, it is fun to observe our own animal's instinct and what their first sense is on board when they become aware of something or someone different.

While the third eye holds the ability to see the unseen, it is also the opportunity to understand the foundation of perception. Being quiet and observing how our own animals are perceiving the world can truly help us understand on a deeper level how they operate in day-to-day life.

7

THE SEVENTH CHAKRA—TRUST

"The Crown Chakra, your crown of holy connection to the Divine, sits at the top of your head, a bright violet disk of light that emanates what we call the Violet Ray of compassionate and protective light. When your Crown Chakra is open and functioning well, you feel intimately aware of your connection to God/Source/Creator energy. When it is blocked or inactive, you feel disconnected from the Divine, and unsure of your relationship to God/Source/Creator."

—Athena Perrakis, Ph.D., *The Ultimate Guide to Chakras: The Beginner's Guide to Balancing, Healing, and Unblocking Your Chakras for Health and Positive Energy*

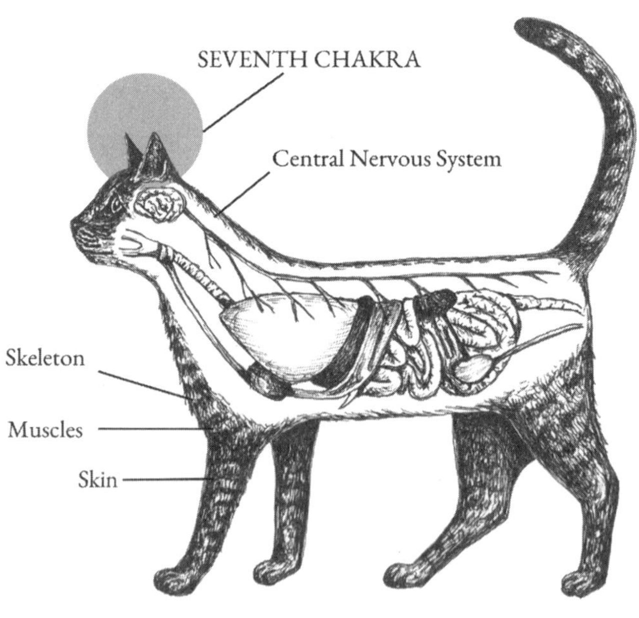

Fig. 8: The seventh chakra (crown chakra)

Here's How We Fly Off a Cliff—Deep Trust, Faith, Interconnectedness, and Finding Purpose

Every year, whether it was when I lived in Carnation, Washington on beautiful acreage, or here in the hills of Santa Clarita, I have experienced something quite magical and loud. Raven Flight School. It goes something like this, mom and dad are swooping elegantly by their fledglings who dot the branches in the distance. The parents effortlessly do a figure eight or infinity sign and let out an encouraging caw. The swaying branches with little black raven dots can hardly hold the enthusiasm. I picture the mom and dad smiling and saying, "See? You can do this." The fledglings who barely have all their wing and tail feathers in, scream back. I always imagine one of them calling, "Wow, come back." Another might say, "I can't do that," and the next one might say, "Watch me, watch me," but he can't leave the branch.

Over the next few weeks, I see them all make left turns in the air. Then they all make right turns. I can tell the difference between the graceful wing strokes of the parents and the fledglings trying so hard. Sometimes the parents use my backyard for "here's how we fly off a cliff." In no time they are almost the same size as the parents, but I know who the kids are by the open mouth waiting for that bit of food. Each bite is delivered with care and assurance from their parents. At the end of the day, I hear the little guttural sounds as if they are all saying "move over" as they squeeze into the nest and get settled into the nest for the night. Raven flight school starts again early the next morning.

Even though they are built to fly—and they are simply activating stored DNA that comes with the package they incarnated into in this lifetime called: raven—it is still an act of faith and trust to take a leap from that safe, though precariously bouncing branch, for the first time. And what faith and trust it must take for those parents to say, "It's time to leave the nursery."

Surely science would say it is simply instinct. But faith would have to play a role in why those clutching little feet would release their grip, open their wings, and jump.

While faith and instinct seem contradictory, faith may be as fundamental as instinct for animals.

The seventh chakra, for all, is the top of the head. It is considered the connection to the divine as if there is a golden cord from the top of the head going straight up to the heavens. The seventh chakra is also pure, unadulterated faith in existence. Animals don't intellectualize their connection to the divine; it just is. For the most part, they start out grounded and divinely connected at the same time.

Our animals at home demonstrate what we love to call "unconditional love," as if we are the deity or represent Spirit to them. There is a devotion. Which is, in part, what draws us to animals. I don't believe that animals are all unconditional. At my house, I have daily proof to the contrary, my animals are quite conditional! Either way, we are drawn in by the purity of spirit that animals exhibit, their loyalty and joy regardless of whether it's a sunny day, the paycheck came in, or the property tax is due in a few days. We are forever in awe of the knowingness and devotion to Spirit in animals.

In good faith or not so good faith, belief or not belief, spiritual or not, it doesn't matter. Most domesticated animals still act as if they have faith in us. And that translates as trust. And those are the tenets of spirituality.

One of my favorite quotes from one of my favorite books is:

> "To me mindfulness is very much like the Holy Spirit. Both are agents of healing. When you have mindfulness, you have love and understanding, you see more deeply, and you can heal the wounds in your own mind. The Buddha was called the King of Healers. In the Bible, when someone touches Christ, he or she was healed. It is not just touching a cloth that brings about a miracle. When you touch deep understanding and love, you are healed."
>
> ——*Living Buddha, Living Christ,* Thich Nhat Hanh

The Question of Faith, Religion, and Spirituality

Jane Goodall has seen chimpanzees weave joyously over a waterfall—she called it the waterfall dance. Scientists have tried to cancel out ritualized behavior as any type of spirituality. Yet, Jane Goodall would argue that if the definition of spirituality is the experience of appreciating magnificent, unknowable powers at work beyond us—and she has seen animals in the wild experience awe and wonder—why wouldn't they then also have feelings of some kind of spirituality?

Spirit is defined as a non-physical part of a being, the emotions, character, and soul. It is believed to remain once the body has died.

Spirit is also a quality or element of a person or animal. For example, I have always loved "spirited" horses, I have lived with many. I define it as "spicy curiosity."

Spirit is also a ghost. Or booze.

Spirituality has two defining characteristics:

1. A belief in something much bigger than us —and faith in life itself.
2. Sacred meaning while finding purpose.

Most animals aren't laying on their back staring at the stars and pondering the meaning of life. Yet, I have communicated with animals who are very philosophical, it's part of their essence, their nature. They are observant, surmising, some may even be judgmental (more cats!), and they are seeking.

Taking this a step further and asking, "Do they have a belief in religion?" The answer is no on the surface but—if religion by definition is: cultural systems, behaviors, practices, morals, ethics, worldview of the supernatural, transcendence, and spiritual elements—we can't say no entirely.

We do see animals fully engage in cultural systems, behaviors, morals, and their own set of ethics of the pack, pride, herd, or flock. Some do have a sense of the supernatural. Many people have experienced their animals having an awareness of the presence of the animal or person who has passed.

It's not my job to prove it to you, but I hope you do ponder and witness on your own.

Because, we have all seen the spirit of an animal shine through as they embody an experience, they are fully engaged in the activity without a single thought. The zone. We have all seen animals in purpose and have a sense of their reverence for the activity, even down to the dog digging in the yard!

If this isn't inspired, then I don't know what is:

- Hawks rising up, wings fully spread and soaring up and down while playing on the thermals, as a surfer would ride a wave.
- Horses running for fun and kicking their heels up, getting everyone else riled up into that energy.
- A cat running through the house after a good poop (okay that might be more of a physical pleasure than spiritual!).

- Dogs completely in a zone when they play.
- Being in a zone with our animal companions.
- Baby elephants rolling in mud as if it were heaven itself.
- Baby zebras running and playing.
- A male African weaver industriously preparing a nest to meet the woman of his dreams and show off the beautiful home he has created.
- Big cats to domestic cats grooming themselves.
- A bear getting into a pond after a long hot day.

And even in the more serious moments:

- Elephants who return a year later to the bones of one of their deceased loved ones.
- A male hornbill gently passing food beak to beak to his wife to feed their babies, then standing guard over the hole in the tree where they reside.

Inspiration means "in spirit"—being inspired by a divine force.

I would say that animals are spiritual, and to what degree depends on the individual itself. Just like humans.

According to Merriam Webster, faith is a firm belief in something of which there is no proof. Complete trust. And while this chakra embodies that concept, our animals personify this with us daily.

Forgiveness is a biblical commandment and considered a virtue.

The gray whale was hunted nearly to extinction in the mid 1800s and again in the early 1900s all over the world. Their blubber was sought after. They are completely extinct in areas where they once thrived. In California and Mexico, they were easily targeted because of their migration habit of going down to Mexico to the warm waters to create a nursery and back up to Alaska in late March or April. Plus, the mamas and their babies really hug the coastline and try to swim through the kelp beds for protection, if possible.

The Sea of Cortez in Mexico has become a mecca for these whales, there are pregnant whales, whales hoping to get pregnant, and mommas, babies, and lots of juveniles. It's like the whole party ends up in Mexico for spring break. Much like the humpback migration from Alaska to Maui, that little bay becomes a crib, and they have a whale of a time!

While these gray whales have every reason to want nothing to do with us humans, their collective memory could kick in as they slowly rebuild their population. Rather, they go up to the boats in these little villages in Mexico. Not only do they go up to the boats to be petted, but they also send their babies to the people. It has become a destination activity in the ecotourism world, kissing whales.

Mustangs who have been taken away from their entire family in violent roundups with helicopters, chaos, and mean humans, often find a home with a human. Most will eventually drop their defenses and slowly settle into life with a domestic herd of horses, dogs, cats, and humans.

Horses in general have endured a heavy load (literally) from us. Cows who have their babies taken away every year still look on with kindness, albeit a sad kindness. Dogs and horses have gone to war, sun bears and moon bears sit for humans to pull their bile out, we eat animals (I don't), we set them up to fight for entertainment, and we have them entertain us in the equivalent of a bathtub.

And yet, they forgive us. Some animals are even altruistic. Humpbacks have been called "altruistic" as they will take on a pod of orcas going after seals, other fish, gray whale babies, other humpbacks, and more. Many animals in sanctuaries who, once they overcome their own wounding, will become friends with other animals of different species, all relating to the fact that they are finally safe.

The Gentle Barn in Santa Clarita, California, and Tennessee, has countless stories of animals being able to be ambassadors for humans who are mentally, physically, and emotionally wounded. Once animals settle in at the Gentle Barn, they can become part of programs for inner city youths, veterans, former drug addicts, and more. They have had horrible trauma and yet, they turn around and offer kindness to a strange human. I am so grateful to be close to one of the founders, Ellie Laks, and be part of communicating and using healing modalities for their animals. They are truly doing miracles on this planet.

The Sheldrick Wildlife Trust: Haven for Elephants and Rhinos in Kenya is another miraculous center as I mentioned in Chapter 2. They are the leaders in integrating orphan elephants into the wild. Elephants are orphaned because of human–wildlife conflict; occasionally because of a wildlife attack, or poaching.

Seventh Chakra Symbolism

In the 30 years I have been working with animals, no one has ever called me over because of a religious war between two dogs in a household. Animals aren't competitive over their divine connection, though they can have resource or territory battles.

The seventh chakra is the portal to the divine—trust, faith, our ability to feel connected to God/Universe/Source/Spirit.

Faith, belief, and Spirit are all things that have created wars for time immemorial. Some humans have a lot of wounding and trauma about belief, faith, and religion.

Pegasus, the ancient being that was here to take us to the heavens, has been grounded and we are here to take that relationship and make it heavenly.

Seventh Chakra Species-Specific/Wild and Domestic

The top of the head is not just a center of connection to the Divine; it also represents an animal's faith—in us and in other beings.

Sometimes we are simply the agent, the shepherd for their eternal connection. Just like the above story about the recovering orphans of the Sheldrick Wildlife Trust, animals return with their injured or sick friends back to the camp for the humans to help. For some animals, in the collective DNA, we have helped. And we have created a sense of trust and the ability to care for them.

When we humans do good, we usually do great.

Caring for animals dates back to when we domesticated them. It wasn't all utilitarian, even though they were working animals. In ancient times and throughout the medieval area, there was companionship and love.

Husbandry (the care, breeding, and cultivation of crops and animals) was all-encompassing back in the day. There weren't veterinarians. People had to take things into their own hands. And once veterinary care came into being, not everyone could afford it.

Modern veterinary care came out of what would be considered today, witch doctors, magic potions, quackery, and all the things I have spent the last 30 years working with and teaching about: energy healing. Although, 3,000 years ago, doctors in China did acupuncture on horses. They were considered "horse priests."

Meanwhile, in Mesopotamia, two types of "doctors" were manifesting: *asu*—the medical doctor who treated illness or injury, based on observation; and *asipu*—faith healers, who used magical incantations, herbs, and prayer. Both types of doctors were interchangeable for humans and animals. Both were seen as necessary.

Simultaneously, this was developing with the Greeks, Romans, Indians, and Egyptians (who loved their animals). These cultures also similarly used doctors and healers together to treat conditions and illness for both animals and humans.

A lot of these cultures believed that illness was a supernatural event or punishment from the powers that be, and Hippocrates came along and said, no. And he showed the world that eating well, exercise, baths, massage, aromatherapy, and mood elevating activities were the keys to health. I couldn't have said it better myself.

Back to the history of helping animals . . .

There was a period in history during which the medieval church did not care about pets. Animals were partners, slaves, transportation, and/or food. Then, one day, in the mid 1300s, the church recognized the benefits to the health of humans when they had animal companionship and something to care for.

But not everyone could afford a doctor, so help for animals was still in the form of magic words, rituals, potions, incantations, faith, tradition, and not-so-modern science. Basically, modern veterinary medicine came out of healers who consulted the stars, called upon saints and holy figures, repeated incantations (in Latin, Hebrew, or gibberish), charms, tied holy objects to animals' necks, sprinkled holy water with sacred words, and a sprinkled some of emerging science on the side. Islamic "doctors" used incantations, signs, symbols, and numerology.

What we now know of as veterinary medicine came on board somewhere in the mid 1700s.

The Shadow Side of the Seventh Chakra

The shadow side of this chakra is the disconnection from the divine. Throughout history, the natural world was part of the fabric of everyday life as well as being revered as part of the divine. Shamans, priests, and priestesses brought the unseen to light and because much of spirituality included nature and wildlife, it was represented, it had meaning, it was relevant to look at a "totem."

As time went on, we have felt disconnected from nature and wildlife, as a result, we are disconnected from an aspect of divinity.

Separation is an illusion because we can never be separated from the divine, or nature for that matter.

Yet, years of unhealthy theology didn't help. The idea of man being created in the image of God took on a distortion and dominion that put us on the top of the pyramid, and everything else was simply serving us.

When it comes to people who "love animals" it seems the pendulum swings either direction on our love for animals and doesn't stop in the middle. People can love animals so much that they have devalued any self-love, seeing our own divine nature, or the human contribution to the planet. The swing to the other side is cognitive dissonance about playing with your dog at home and hunting on the weekend with your friends. And even one step further, the cognitive dissonance of being an animal lover and eating them.

The first group will stop when they see a hawk and Google "what does hawk mean." We have objectified and commodified their existence, rather than taking the moment in to really see who the hawk is, and what they are up to.

I can be on one of my Facebook lives and sharing that a road runner just ran by the window and the comments in the feed will light up with everyone asking, "Oh, what does that mean?" I always say, "It means a road runner just ran by my window."

I say that because at some point, the hawk flying or the road runner running by my window is spiritual enough and is every day.

I watch people come into my program starting out as animal lovers and graduate from the program as animal communicators or energy healers and I would call them animal people. They may have started out with reaching hands, needing to touch and make cooing noises over every single animal, and graduate into a sense of "I see you" appreciation.

On my wildlife trips, we do a certain meditation that involves bringing our nervous system down and moving into deep waves of appreciation. Appreciation holds a different quality than love or gratitude. Appreciation has love and gratitude in it but isn't transactional. It stands on its own in the distance as a recognition and sensitivity to the magnitude, quality, significance, admiration, and value of something.

To appreciate someone or something allows them to have full agency.

Ted Andrews in his wonderful book, *Animal Speak: The Spiritual & Magical Powers of Creatures Great and Small* (Llewellyn Publications, 1993) says:

> "There was a time when humanity recognized itself as part of nature, and nature as part of itself. Dreaming and waking were inseparable realities, the natural and the supernatural merged and blended. People used images of nature to express this unity and to instill a transpersonal kind of experience."

Beautiful.

So, do animal oracle decks have significance or relevance? Yes, of course, if they are sought after for reflection and symbolism.

But when we don't connect with nature—speaking theoretically as our modern culture—we have lost touch with nature within. When we've lost touch with nature within, we have lost our agency. Then we over-identify with the bear card we pulled and then we wait for our subconscious awakening because that's what the card says it means, or hibernation because that's what bears do and we go on needing something, someone, to tell us what to do.

In this isolation . . . when we feel as though we must be saved, we need salvation, and so we identify with those who we think need to be saved and need salvation. Through our own disconnected empathic lens, we see only the "other" suffering. And to save ourselves, we must save others.

While rescuing animals is a noble thing to do, when it is done from this unhealed, fractured part of ourselves, the identification with the "rescue" continues. While healing often comes from this—and this is maybe the first point of contact with nature—imagine if we started from the position of being connected with nature, wildlife, and the divine.

Even in conservation circles, people rush to see that one near-extinct apex predator and forget about all the other animals that may be facing extinction.

We forget from our shared and connected divinity within, that we are interdependent with the animal beings, and when they're gone, we're gone too.

Seventh Chakra Emotions and Energetics

If the top of the head is the physical representation of this chakra connecting to the divine, and animals have had experiences where they have had head injuries, it is no mystery why they don't trust and, in particular, why they don't trust a human hand coming at them.

In many ways we represent the Divine to them, so when human hands have hurt this area, an animal's trust in the Divine is shattered. This is an important place to work with to help animals recover their sense of faith in the world.

Faith has a feeling. I have faith the sun will come up. I don't question that. Animals don't either. When that feeling is not present, there is zero stability.

Dr. Jaak Panksepp did extensive research on neuroscience and behavior. He was an Estonian-American neuroscientist and psychobiologist who coined the term "affective neuroscience."

The reason I bring him up is because his position is that we, and animals, have feelings because they tell us what supports, and what detracts from, our survival. Dr. Panksepp identified the core emotion systems that animals have (and that we share), calling them the blue ribbon emotions, because they:"generate well-organized behavior sequences that can be evoked by localized electrical stimulation of the brain." This means that when you stimulate the brain systems for one of the core emotions, you always get the same behaviors from the animal.

The blue ribbon emotions systems are seeking, play, care, panic, lust, fear, and rage.

If you've ever been hit in the head or hit your head, you may meet the term head on: blind rage. It is like you don't know who to blame and come out swinging.

Animals experience this as well. Not only that, in their quadrupedal bodies, the compensation pattern may in fact continue to contribute to the old head injury or, stress can make the head feel like it is going to explode and bam, the dog bites, the horse bucks, and/or the cat strikes. Add in the vantage point of dogs and cats being below us, and looking up, completely vulnerable, and horses not sure where to look and focus.

We humans don't even see it coming because we don't have the understanding from an emotional/physical perspective, nor are we tracking body language.

If you have ever had an animal communication reading or a medical intuition scan on your animal, then you will start to notice the quick build up like a freeze-frame sequence. You will see the back freeze, the head tilt, and the action happen. There will be five subtle signs that for that animal are like screaming neon.

A horse trainer, Anna, called me because she couldn't figure out Arnie. He was a tall thoroughbred. She purchased him for her riding academy where kids get to experience having a horse of their own without their parents having to make a significant financial investment. It is often a gentle precursor to purchasing a horse. Arnie would be someone who kids could fall in love with.

Except he had a mean buck.

When I communicated with Arnie, I sensed a very good guy, a bit lost, a guy who wanted that one-on-one connection, and a big confusion. He knew people fell in love with him because on the ground, he was sweet as apple pie. He was aware that he had big rolling gaits, the kind of ride that people under twenty can learn on and the people over fifty crave.

But there was a point, usually moving into the left lead canter, where it went haywire. Just to back up, when a horse leads to the left in the canter, the hind drops like a coil, lifts the front end and strikes off from the right hind. His experience in that moment is a full-on head explosion. And here is why.

First of all, it felt like in one of his prior jobs—likely the time he was a polo horse—he had an incident where he jammed his right hind from a slide and a hard stop. That jam went from the lower hind, up into the hip. It constricted the mid back on the right side and withers (between the shoulders). Which then shut off the left shoulder. But the right side of the withers was sending a reverberating "uh oh" to the cervical vertebrae (C1 and C2), which made the head explode with noise and chaos, almost making him dizzy. All from the original pain.

Now, do I feel like he is in pain now? No, I feel like there is discomfort, scar tissue, minimal loss of range of motion, and a big muscle memory of what has happened in the past. So, in order to avoid it, we will ditch the rider.

Because in general, he loves connection, approval, and is so sweet in his essence. The violent way in which he ejects riders can only be from pain, or the fear of pain.

The brain is built to protect. Like animals, humans are still protecting from the original caveman life. We haven't archetypally readjusted the brainwaves to "wow, life is super easy." Instead, we still have suspicion lurking. This is how conspiracy theories are built. This is muscle memory. This is "the sky is falling."

Unless we have retrained the brain or addressed the muscle memory, the brain will keep firing off.

And in the case of Arnie, exploding.

Seventh Chakra Organs, Structure, Body Parts, and Meridians

Organs

The seventh, or crown, chakra sits at top of the head in humans and animals. It governs the entire skeletal and muscular system, cerebral cortex, central nervous system, peripheral nervous system (PNS), neocortex, fascia, and skin.

- Physiological systems at work here: Skeletal (supports body), muscular (holds skeleton together, posture, and mobility), dermatology (protection of everything), central nervous system (command center of everything), and homeostasis!
- Endocrine systems at work here: Thalamus (the communicator—everything is processed through here before it is sent to different parts of the brain, nervous system and/or organs).
- Nerve plexus: Central nervous system (CNS) and peripheral nervous system (PNS). CNS integrates the received information and coordinates and influences all for the activity for all the body parts!
- Spine/Skeleton: Top of Skull, cervical vertebrae, joints, and neurocranium bones (or cranial bones) that protect the brain. There are: 22 bones in the human head, 34 bones in a horse head; 50 bones in a dog head; and 29 bones in a cat head.
- Proprioception: Body movement, position, balance.

Meridians and Traditional Chinese Medicine

Governing Vessel (GV), Triple Heater (TH), Gallbladder (GB), and Bladder (BL).

So many meridians cross over the top of the head. In this chapter we have had a heavy focus on the stress that would come from a head injury, we must also balance the information out with the calming of the top of the head if someone is not traumatized. Governing Vessel 20 (top of head) is known to calm and relieve stress and anxiety.

Putting It All Together: It's Not Just Skin Deep

- Fascia, think of fascia as the top sheet under the skin. If there has been an accident, and the sheet is wrinkled, this is considered soft tissue damage, and can definitely inhibit mobility.

- Skin issues and conditions.
- The bones in the head are joined together by sutures which are like fibrous joints. While it is believed in scientific communities that the only moveable bone is the mandible, if you've ever seen a horse, dog, or cat with the slightest imbalance of where their eyes sit, they have likely had a head injury, and this can shift their sight.
- The nervous system is responsible for processing sensory information, this includes neural pathways, sensory neurons, and the brain, perception, and interoception.
- Perception integrates stimuli from the senses and experience in the external world, creating awareness.
- Interoception is sensing the internal—from cells to bones to organs, to hormones, and even the immune response. It is our physiology at work, and it facilitates homeostasis and self-awareness. But that self-awareness and homeostasis is not a self-awareness where we say "Oh, my liver is talking to me" (though that is possible). Interoception is more like the autonomic nervous system, it just works. We don't have to think about breathing or blinking, it just is.

Stories

Time

Time could be considered a deep-seated belief system. We have no idea if it really exists and yet it is something that we have imposed upon ourselves probably deeper than anything. Sometimes if I'm late I feel that I can stretch time or in other situations I feel I've compressed time, but it is so anchored in by so many minds, this is a hard one to bend.

So, the animals go right along with us. Foo is the cat of a friend of mine, Polly. Polly had asked me to feed Foo twice a day while she was out of town. They had just moved into a new place and a friendly face was crucial.

On Sunday morning I stopped by Foo's house very early to feed her. I was wearing my riding clothes, ready to go out to see my horse. When I walked in there was no Foo in sight. I looked amidst the boxes, no Foo. I looked in every closet, no Foo. I was beside myself. I then noticed a window where she had pushed open the screen.

I sat on the bed and as quiet as one could do so in a panic, in a telepathic scream I checked in with Foo: "Where are you?"

"I'm fine, I'm fine, I'm fine, I'll be home at 6:00." "What?" That's all I got from her. That was nearly 12 hours away. I went out and saw folks in their Sunday best leaving for church. "Have you seen a cat that looks like . . . ?"

One elderly gentleman had seen her cut through his backyard. So, there I am in riding clothes cutting through people's backyards in Los Angeles. I gave up and went to the barn. I came back and this time I got quiet again. "I'll be back at 6:00."

I still wasn't taking that as a legitimate answer and started knocking on doors. I handed out my cards to folks saying, "If you see her, call me. I'll come right back over." As you might expect, when I handed my card to one sassy woman she said, "You're an animal communicator, why don't you just tell her to come back?"

I explained nicely that animals have free will, you don't just tell them what to do but that Foo had told me she'd be back at six.

I gave up my search and went home. At 5:45 I went back to Foo's house. I opened the front door and who should be sitting proudly in the entryway? Why Foo, of course, in her full glory with a meow as if to say, "I told you I'd be home by 6:00."

I couldn't resist telling the neighbor that Foo had gotten home on time, after I nailed shut all of the screens.

Ravi

CWALU (Communication With All Life University) offers advanced training for animal communication and energy healing. In the Advanced Animal Communication (Level 3), Behavior, Relationships, and Dynamics, the students communicate with animals who have a challenge— either emotional, behavioral, relationship, or physical. In this class, it is my opportunity to help the soon to be animal communicators finesse their readings.

The dog we were connecting with, Ravi, is cared for by one of the students in the school, Tina. Tina shared that the dog snaps at people when they reach down to touch him. He's super cute so everyone wants to pet him. To top it all off, Tina lives in an ashram so there are a lot of animal-loving people around.

The students got loud and clear how serious this dog is. When he puts his emotional support vest on, it is like he has done a spit and polish on his outfit so the world could see how invested he is in his job. He would not be one for small talk, he is all business, and very deep. They did an amazing job.

Upon further investigation into the animal medical intuition scan, it was pretty evident that there was something going on in his head and neck. One person got that he felt like his eyes would be poked out when the hand came near him. Nearly everyone talked about the tension in his neck. I kept getting an image of being a puppy and face planting, and that the neck vertebrae were compressed. Tina said he faceplanted all of the time as a puppy because his head was so much bigger than his body and he would topple over in his food bowl, the water dish, and more.

Then I had Tina slowly go over and do a temperature gauge of his head and neck so she (as the client) could see for herself where in fact the discomfort was, and why he would want to protect his head from people touching him. There was heat between the eyes and varying degrees of warmth throughout the rest of the head and neck. It was clear for Tina that massage or chiropractic would help.

Ravi doesn't have to become anything different than he is, but comfort is on the way! Not all dogs (or many dogs) want to be touched on the head by a stranger, even if they don't have protection issues.

Olivia

Olivia was my soul mate dog who did my life with me for 14 and a half years. About six years into our life together after a whole lot of losses, we ended up with Isabella, a beautiful black lab who was basically feral. Isabella had been a client, I acquired her from a wonderful rescue shelter after communicating with her for the rescue. She was a foster fail that lasted an hour.

But she was so terrified of everything, and especially blond women. At the time, I had a little healing center going and the people whose horses I was boarding were blond women. The terror that coursed through her body and detonated in her brain was like nothing I'd ever seen. If I introduced a leash, she screamed as if she were being tortured. They had to drug her to bring her to me.

I finally figured out that she trusted Olivia. She was never going to trust me if I kept trying things. I became "pressure." So, I employed Olivia in the dog training. Olivia and I loved training. We had done obedience, agility, sheep herding, and more.

I would say to Isabella, "Watch the video." Then I would introduce the word "sit." Olivia would sit. Isabella would watch Olivia and then sit. We learned "down" this way. I eventually was able to put the leash on Isabella after watching the video of me putting the leash on Olivia.

I got Isabella on September eighteenth. My first book was coming out in November, and I was going to have a workshop at my place at the end of January, with people coming in from all over the country. I had so many trainers try to help me. Not only did they think that my goal of end of January for Isabella to be able to be in the same house as strangers was unrealistic, but they also gave up on training in general. In many ways, I literally trained the most terrified dog I'd ever met through Olivia. Eventually, she listened to me and trusted me through Olivia. I always say that I learned a ton about dog training with Olivia, but I learned about behavior with Isabella. She was my soul mate teacher dog.

Not only was she okay for that workshop the following January, but she also eventually became the greeter at every one of my workshops. And she'd especially love you if you had a sandwich in your bag.

THE EIGHTH CHAKRA— THE ECOSYSTEM, MORPHIC RESONANCE, AND YOUR HOME

"Morphic resonance takes place through morphogenetic fields and indeed gives rise to their characteristic structures. Not only does a specific morphogenetic field influence the form of a system, but also the form of this system influences the morphogenetic field and through it becomes present to subsequent similar systems."

—RUPERT SHELDRAKE, *Morphic Resonance: The Nature of Formative Causation*

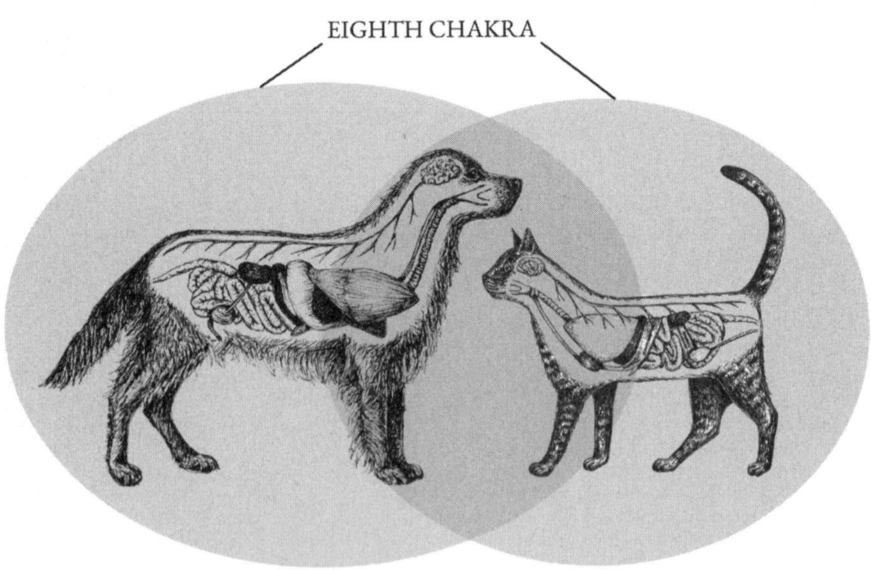

Fig. 9: The eighth chakra (brachial chakra)

Heaven on Earth—
Setting the Thermostat to Harmony

I love a good ghost tour. I've done a ghost tour in some cool places, but the one in Charleston, South Carolina stands out. We started in the graveyard (of course) and walked through the historic part of town.

The guide was excellent. In the first brick building that we went to, a murder had taken place. Several people were blamed. As the guide shared the high drama of the old tale, he also shared that when such an event like a murder happens, all of the feelings get stuck in the wall. In other words, even if you don't believe in "ghosts" per se, the walls hold the experience.

Bricks are porous. Brick was once mud, and clay can absorb water. And emotions. Wood is porous. It was once a living being that also could absorb water. And emotions. Cement comes from minerals that were all once vibrant. Just because these materials don't seem alive today, in their current incarnation, as buildings and furniture, they are vibrating at a different frequency, yet they still absorb all.

Naturally, if something terrible happens in a room, the walls could tell the story. Equally, the room could hold joy. And that is why people are drawn to churches, temples, and ashrams, they hold the energy of faith and trust.

The space itself holds energy, but also, the beings that occupy the space can shape the energy. The field of energy is made up of our energy fields that we each bring to the party.

Dr. Rupert Sheldrake wrote a book called *Dogs That Know When Their Owners Are Coming Home: And Other Unexplained Powers of Animals* (Crown, 2011) and had set up an experiment in London where there were time-stamped cameras placed at home, and at the office or workplace of participants. Everyone left their work at odd times as opposed to the time when they normally did. In each instance, the camera at home showed the dog getting up and going to the door to wait for their person to come home.

He introduced the theory of a morphic field. Basically, a morphic field is an organized database of information in the form of the electromagnetic field that holds activities, thoughts, beliefs, and behaviors. He suggests that information or memory is transmitted through an invisible field, rather than physical mechanisms. He expanded his theory to say that this morphic resonance creates a collective pattern of behavior based on the pattern of a group's field. Each species has its own morphic resonance, as does each individual. The combined field is unique.

Excerpted from my second book, *Energy Healing for Animals*:

> "When we speak of animals as mirrors of ourselves, it's morphic resonance we're describing. The morphic field we create with our animals has a pattern of its own that influences everything within it. It also has a memory, and its influence extends beyond time and space. It has a like-attracts-like pattern, which is to say that we draw energies to our morphic field that are similar to our own energies. And anything that doesn't jibe with our field feels 'uncomfortable.'"

Emotional leadership is the way of setting the energetic, morphic tone, like setting the thermostat. I always say let's set the thermostat to Harmony!

An ecosystem is another way of saying morphic resonance, and vice versa.

On one of the last days in Ol Pejeta Conservancy in central Kenya, we came upon a scene that I will never forget. We slowly drove into a valley that had a pastoral feel to it. Zebras were playfully bucking or grazing with every type of antelope that lives in Kenya. Muddy Cape buffalo emerged from the waterhole as the elephants slowly approached. All the tails of all of the species seemed choreographed as they swished flies away in unison. It was heaven. It reminded me of what Eden must be like.

Whether myth, allegory, or truth, the Garden of Eden before the fall would have been my version of heaven on earth. There were no predators or prey, just animals and humans being together.

With the "fall of man," or the birth of ego came the suspicion, the fear, the shame, a division between good and bad, right and wrong, better or worse, stronger or weaker, victim or victor, evil or pious and all the things we can create an "or" around. The oneness, the one-mind was gone. And if the resonance was to reflect that, we now see the evolution of predation at every level at every turn.

Yet, beings come together and work together in herds, packs, prides, colonies, flocks, murders, and more. They create their morphic resonance or ecosystem where they are communicating within their own species-specific ecosystem.

Working together within the same species:

- Elephants
- Lions
- Chimpanzees
- Wolves
- Dolphins
- Orcas

And then we see that expanded ecosystem where animals are cooperating from different species.

Working together as many species:

- Cattle and egrets, and horses and egrets. When I lived in Florida, my horses had "friends."
- Remora (fish) that are found on dolphins, sharks, and whales.
- Humpbacks saving seals from transient orcas.
- Antelope, zebras, wildebeest, and giraffes all graze together.
- Oxpeckers on rhinos have made a good deal. Because rhinos have such poor sight and great hearing, they just blaze ahead in ramming mode based on the sound of the oxpecker.
- Henry (cat) and Isabella (dog) counter-surfing in my kitchen. Cat knocks everything off, dog has a buffet.

Eighth Chakra Symbolism

The eighth chakra in the Kundalini world is white and is believed to be all about the aura, the energy field that surrounds you, and your subtle body. This field of energy filters everything that comes into your field. Your field senses the environment and knows whether it is contributing to your health or well-being. Everything that becomes your biology or reality comes into your field first.

Animals have an awareness of this and the connection to the other within this field of energy. Our aura and electromagnetic field of energy (and combined, collective field with the others—the morphic resonance) is the first line of defense for protection from challenging energies.

This field of energy has resonance across time and space and holds our records, the imprint of this moment in time, as well as the individual and collective soul record, the Akashic Records. Instead of genetic inheritance alone, species inherit a "memory" of their predecessors' behaviors or structures through a universal field. It attracts the familiars back to us who may have reincarnated in the form of our animals. And us to them.

Eighth Chakra Species-Specific/Wild and Domestic

When I describe that idyllic Eden moment in Kenya, I'm also reminded of how peace and strength in numbers created a unified field. I still talk about it with the people who went on that trip. A few of my guests returned with me on a trip to Zimbabwe and had a similar experience at a watering hole in Mana Pools. It was hard to eat lunch with all of the activities of the wildlife around. And the elephants that came right up to the waterhole a little later.

Peace easily gets pierced once the hunt is on and chaos ensues. The morphic resonance becomes part of survival. If the predator(s) are a collective (lions, wolves, cheetahs, orcas), then they are in their own oneness (morphic resonance) as they maneuver together without words to take down their prey. Prey struggles to stay in their own collective communication as there is safety in numbers.

The pressure of the predator is not released until the predator is gone. So, the field of energy has either the fight or flight pressure, chaos feel, or the rest and digest peaceful feel. Pressure and release.

The Shadow Side of the Eighth Chakra

It is hard to make a good decision when we can feel the chaos of fight or flight. Seeking, curiosity, and play are out of the window when we are feeling sad, mad, or scared.

Also, this field of energy can sense when there are too many things in the environment that are attacking our system, and that includes all non-native EMFs from technology, combined with preservatives and other questionable ingredients in foods and our water supply, and many factors which contribute to fight or flight. The polarity (balance) can be thrown off easily. Being in this state long term can eventually overwhelm and tax the system.

Eighth Chakra Emotions and Energetics

Collective consciousness isn't just a phenomenon with wildlife, it is in our homes, it is in our barns, it is in our neighborhoods.

I had a friend, Kelli, who lived on the property with her dogs and her horse in Carnation, Washington. One day Kelli set out on a trail ride. About a half hour after she left, I went to fetch my horses and something (likely a bear) had scared them so much, there was no catching them. They ran like wild mustangs for about half an hour. None of my tricks worked that day and I resorted to going back into the house and drinking coffee.

When Kelli returned a couple of hours later, she said that she had a scary moment when her horse, Doc, was starting to buck. I asked her what time this had happened, and she said about a half hour after she left. I told her that my horses had become unglued and were running like crazy.

Even though she was a mile away with thick woods between us, plenty of sight, sound, and smell buffers between us, Doc was still reacting within that field of energy, miles away.

First Chakra and How It Correlates to the Eighth Chakra

There are so many times that the first chakra is connected to the eighth chakra, that place where the crown and the root meet. It is so apropos in that it is where divine guidance and grounding are put to the test.

Because safety and survival are built into "instinct," animals are used to checking into their field of energy. You might see a nostril activate on your dog at the park and the fur on the flank start to ripple. They are feeling with all senses in all directions. They are tapping into the energy field that is connected to them and provides safety.

We've all done this. As much as I love the tools that I share to stay grounded and divinely connected and everything human in between, I remember two distinct situations where the field of energy was so thick, I had to work overtime. One was 9/11, and the other was the beginning of the Pandemic.

Fear was in the air. Both are situations that, for the first shocking moment, provided such a pivotal connection and opportunity, but were both anchored immediately to a stricken sensibility, an abject terror.

Whether I consciously knew what was happening or not on any given day after those experiences, my body became a GPS for what was happening. I had to cling to my routines of meditation, self-care, exercise, care of my animals, and work.

We have all experienced a connection to the collective. It is truly a beautiful thing. I honestly believe with discipline and creativity we can turn the collective into a true resource of love and nurturing. We can start by creating that sanctuary in our homes and be that resource for our beloved animal companions.

Eighth Chakra Behavior, Dynamics, and Relationships

As tragic as it can be when you have to rehome an animal because they are not getting along with the other animal(s) in the household, often it is because it is not in resonance with the animals who have been living there for years. Even though it is looked down upon by hardcore rescuers, you may very well be doing that animal a favor to find "its forever home" that is in complete resonance with their being.

Eighth Chakra Organs and Systems

While the auric field doesn't have "an" organ it takes care of, it takes care of all organs, glands, structures, systems. It is almost like the protective casing around the body.

Being aware of environmental stressors for your animals can be very important as it can break the system down.

Environmental stressors could be anything from mold to bad neighbors, terrible lighting to emotional pressure, etc.

Animals who are "on" all the time are especially susceptible in this setting.

Putting It All Together: Language and Awareness

Language is a communication system, made up of vocabulary and grammar to best describe a concept or a series of feelings or a movie-like imagery. Language does not exist in the animal kingdom except for our language guiding them. They have their own systems of communication – their various vocalizations, body language, and much other more subtle ways. One of the most important things to recognize is that "language" may come in the form of vibration, frequency, and/or the electromagnetic field. Animals are not only aware of it, but their life also depends upon being tuned into it.

We hear the stories of people running out into the water in Thailand to see why the tide was way out during the tsunami, while the elephants were cutting a path through the jungle to get the hell out of there.

Animals can sense barometric changes, storms, and earthquakes. Tuning into our environment and creating a safe haven with harmony can be just what the energetic doctor ordered!

In some spiritual circles and indigenous cultures, there is an awareness of ley lines. These invisible lines crisscross the globe and can connect fault lines with the pressure of tectonic plates to spiritual and mystical monuments with landforms that are considered natural wonders. Landscapes often invite this intended path. At one time, humans were aware of an etherial force and placed sacred monuments in alignment with the natural phenomena.

Stories

Ravens and Our Ecosystem

The ravens that lived high in a nest on the Carnation property were within eye line of the house. I lived in up on a hill. Between us was the lower pasture, the barn, and the runs for the horses. As I watched the ravens raise their babies, they watched me with kittens who were born on the property, the dogs that doted on the kittens, and the horses I am a slave to. It was like the ravens were part of the family.

They brought me gifts. They would leave half a loaf of French bread in my round pen. The dogs knew it. The minute the door opened to go feed the horses, the dogs raced down to get the bread. I think they thought that I was leaving them gifts in the form of dog bones, when really, with all of the other chores around the farm, I wasn't picking up the dog bones. So, apart from gifting me with bread, the ravens cleaned up the dog bones. Then they started regifting me those bones in the water troughs.

As I traveled the country teaching animal communication, my students would communicate with one of my horses, Anya. Anya would always tell the classes that she liked clean water. For whatever reason, the ravens loved Anya's water trough and they tended to use it, not only for their own drinking but for cleaning their things. In other words, Anya's water trough could get nasty.

So, I added another water trough right next to Anya's on the side of the fence closest to their nest. I told the ravens loudly, "This is your water trough, please leave Anya's water fresh." I only said it once, and I never had to say it again. The ravens only used their own water trough. I still cleaned it!

What was most impressive about this ecosystem we had was that the ravens gave me plenty of time to get the dogs and cats in if coyotes were in the distance. They had a different caw for eagles, which everyone in this ecosystem knew. I would get my cats in, the field was radio-silent and then an eagle, often two, would fly through as if they were given security clearance.

The minute they were off in the distance, the squirrels would get busy again, the volume on the birdsong went to high again, and peace was restored.

Cheyenne

Cheyenne was the perfect companion for Jane as she stopped her world travel in her mid-twenties and tried her hand at a couple careers. Jane and Cheyenne did everything together. I met them both about seven years ago and the bond was so clear then that they were truly not just cosmic soul mates, they did everything together. At that time, we discussed the fact that Cheyenne didn't like other dogs and that she took her issues to the mat with a few dogs. While Cheyenne was always protecting Jane's being and her heart, Jane was always protecting Cheyenne so that an incident wouldn't occur.

At 18 years old, Cheyenne's true nurturing and adventurous essence was taking a fragile turn. Jane hadn't been without Cheyenne breathing near her—really ever since she got her. Getting another dog was scary for two reasons. Jane didn't want to hurt Cheyenne, especially in the final stretch, as she didn't want her to leave hurt. Make no mistake about Cheyenne, as fragile as she seemed on the one hand, she could still muster up energy and take a puppy down. Or at least try.

Yet there seemed to be a turning point for Cheyenne, as if she knew she wanted to clean this karma up in the end—she didn't want to have that be unfinished business.

All of Jane's animals have a signature soul connection—there is some intangible thread that runs through as a theme. Jane found Dean, an English shepherd as handsome as Cheyenne was beautiful. Even though they were completely different breeds—and Cheyenne looked different now in her graceful aging—energetically it was as if they were from the same lineage.

Cheyenne elegantly accepted little Dean for the wild child that he was. If there were days that she was weaker, she let him know from a sitting position what was too much. It was good for her, and there was joy to have this other. Somewhere it was as if she allowed Dean to heal her misgivings about other dogs, and she was glad to know Jane wouldn't be alone.

Ryker

Diane brought Ryker, a very handsome Belgian Tervuren over with hepatocutaneous syndrome, a rare, progressive disease, basically a liver breakdown that has symptoms of dried and crusty scabs around the feet and other skin ailments. Ryker was seven, and had become Diane's life partner, navigating through much of life, especially now as Diane's husband, Ted, had just died from Hepatitis C, after tragically being rejected for a liver transplant. Ted left behind his three children ranging in ages from late teens to mid-20s. His early death was a real challenge for the whole family. Now, Ryker was suffering from a rare liver disease.

In addition to some supplements and healing, I had Diane continue to see him as perfect. The vets were seeing a whole different picture, basically they hadn't had anyone really survive this, especially with the liver counts that Ryker had. Ryker had a quiet sadness in his eyes as well. He had always held himself in a regal way and was so stunning, but now his demeanor was shrinking—as if he were vulnerable and going away.

Between what Diane had just suffered with her husband, the outcome the vets was portraying , and how Ryker was getting smaller by the minute, this was a tall assignment. Especially when the last thing you're going to believe after losing your husband to a twenty-year liver battle is that your dog was going to survive a rare form of liver disease. I kept saying to Diane, "You can't put Ted's story on this. I don't know what this story will be—but it has to be Ryker's story." I suggested that she go to see my friend, Linda Joy, for people energy work to continue to work through the grief of losing Ted.

Within a short amount of time, she had a true miracle. Against all odds, Ryker lived many, many happy years. The turnaround happened right after the work with Linda Joy and releasing the grief. Yes, there were many other factors, the supplements, the visions for him but by working energetically on herself, Diane was able to collapse the story around Ryker that surrounded him with so much disappointment and devastation.

PART TWO

SOLUTIONS

THE CHAKRA SYSTEM

The full chakra systems of cats, dogs, horses, chicken, and humans are depicted on the color plates in this book.

9

TUNING IN TO THEIR CHAKRAS

"As a human being matures and the chakras develop, each represents the psychological patterns evolving in the individual's life. Most of us react to unpleasant experiences by blocking our feeling and stopping a great deal of our natural energy flow. This affects the development and maturation of the chakras, resulting in inhibition of a fully balanced psychological function."

—BARBARA ANN BRENNAN, *Hands of Light: A Guide to Healing Through the Human Energy Field*

The above quote, while about humans can also be said for animals. The difference is that humans at least express it through words with a therapist or a friend. Animals only express through behavior, or misunderstood emotions. So, it is imperative that we at least check in with the chakras through the techniques that follow below. And have a good animal communicator on hand!!

Up until now, we've been assessing from our mind, the chakras are a theory. In the next three chapters we are going to create some ways to assess, and then balance, the chakras. Journaling is fun because you can really create a measurement for the transformation in your animal and your home.

I have created a little Chakra Healing Kit that you can find here: ***https://author.joanranquet.com/animal-chakra-healing/resources***

You are not just looking to heal the chakra but to understand that it is a key to your awareness of the emotional or physiological challenges for your animal/s. You would want to support the emotional and/or physical challenge as best you can and balance the chakras. This way, healing comes about organically.

So, we start with some reflection, journal questions, and get an assessment. These are simply questions. Nobody will judge you, there won't be a test at the end, it's just a way to start pointing in the direction of harmony. And maybe you already have that. Then you don't need to do this. But you might enjoy the process just for drill because it may create some insights.

And think of the questions as much as you can from the animal's perspective when it comes to the questions about them.

• • • • • • •EXERCISE • QUESTIONS ABOUT YOUR ANIMAL • • • • • •

So, before we get chakra-centric here, let's go ahead and create an overall picture of your animal(s).

General questions

1. Does your animal feel adjusted?
2. Does your animal like other animals?
3. Does your animal like people?
4. Do the animals in your home get along with each other?
5. Is there something you could do about it right now if you answered no to question 3?
6. Is your animal thriving with their health?
7. Is there something you could do about it right now if you answered no to question 3?
8. If your animal is in the end-of-life stages, are you getting them the support they need?

FIRST CHAKRA QUESTIONS

As we mention in Chapter 1, there are some fundamental questions to create safety.

1. Is my own world safe and secure?
2. What adjustments do I have to make to provide that for my animals?
3. Did I grow up with an element of chaos?
4. Is the chaos of my childhood so familiar that I have recreated it in my adult life and am subjecting my animals to what I grew up in?
5. This is not my first chakra "survival" experience, it is theirs? How am I supporting their experience?
6. Has my animal ever known safety?
7. Is my animal able to self soothe?
8. Am I providing safety for my animal?

SECOND CHAKRA QUESTIONS

Remember, these are just questions. Some simple questions which could help enlighten as to the behavior, dynamics, and relationships.

1. How many households has this animal been in?
2. How much armor from heartbreak is this animal carrying?
3. How many people have come and gone?
4. How many animals have come and gone?
5. How many animals have taken all the great jobs?

Simple questions for yourself are:

1. Do I feel sorry for this animal?
2. Am I taking their behavior personally?
3. Is there a "job" I could give them that would help them to feel as though they have purpose?
4. Are there ways I've set up an "off" time, away from the others so they can relax?
5. Are they able to self soothe?

THIRD CHAKRA QUESTIONS AND AWARENESS

Awareness in the wild and at home is experienced, even when nobody is looking! Awareness comes in all forms. Does your animal have an opportunity to experience the following (companions, take a moment to answer as if you are your animal):

1. Awareness in nature.
2. Awareness in the home.
3. Awareness in the show ring .
4. Awareness if you are the runt.
5. Awareness if you are part of family (even if you are part of a boarding situation).
6. Awareness of affection and the need to receive and express it (even if your body is too big to fit in the lap anymore).
7. Awareness of the way others treat you.
8. Awareness of boundaries.

And here are some emotional/energetic scenarios that could lead to a breakdown in the third chakra:

1. Animals that have been rehomed repeatedly.
2. Horses that have changed jobs several times.
3. Animals that are newly adopted when the grief of the former animal hasn't quite subsided.
4. The family dog who has watched the kids it helped raise go off to college.
5. Animals that are picked on by other animals.
6. Animals that were not treated kindly in human households and are now scarred by insecurities.
7. The kick-me sign—the animal with the repeated patterns, owner after owner.
8. The stoic animal that won't let on it is in greater pain than it appears to be.

This list represents just a few of the common issues that might drive a breakdown in this area.

Things that you can do that could quickly support an animal who experiences mental, emotional, or physical challenges in the third chakra area include:

1. Recognizing and appreciating whatever job the animal in your household is doing.
2. Reassigning jobs when big changes are made in a household to help the animal retain a sense of security.
3. Letting new animals know that they are loved.
4. Allowing moments for the animal at the bottom of the pecking order to just breathe and be themselves.
5. Finding activities that help the animal gain a strong sense of self and its relationship with you.

6. Allowing the animal to express itself through play and other joyful activity.
7. Playing with archetypes, assigning a new purpose.
8. Training.
9. Boundaries.
10. Exercise, play, laughing, good food, and clean water to support the animal's health.

And some of the things that enhance their lifestyle and create confidence and healthy self-esteem:

1. Nutrition—a healthy balanced diet for all life!
2. Lifestyle—having a happy lifestyle can include activities that the animal loves to do, as having animals as companions on activities you love to do. Some dogs like to go along for the ride so to speak and that can be a great adventure!
3. Exercise—like humans, exercise plays a key role in an animal's mental, physical, and emotional health.
4. Seeking—finding ways for our animals to be able to seek, whether it is sniffing out in the yard, going on an exploration through the trails, animals need to have their curiosity piqued. If they are homebodies, hide the treats!
5. Training—this is one of the most important things you can do to help an animal be able to have a common language with you. It is not only confidence building but can have a safety factor to it. If your animals aren't trained and someone else had to evacuate your house, what would happen?
6. Management—many people are in a situation where they must manage animals through crate-and-rotate, or keep them in other

rooms, because there has been a bloody dispute. This is not the end of the world, rather a safety measure. As long as all of the parties get a little "me" time with their person or other animals, sometimes this is the best way to keep animals safe and in their confidence.

7. Animal Communication—I can't even tell you how many times animals have been adopted in shelters after an animal communication session because their essence has been revealed. Everyone heals when they feel acknowledged, their story has been told, and they are seen for who they are. This is the gift of animal communication that we can share with others..
8. Energy Healing—this is a very important way of helping an animal to get out of rage or to shut down to be able to be in their body and be who they are.
9. Relationships—Animals like and need each other. Humans are okay but they need to be with the same species. Sometimes even the same breed. When my border collie sees other working dogs, she goes crazy in a great way.
10. Role models—sometimes your more feral animals need to see it through another animal. A feral cat may settle in faster with another cat. Mustangs need to watch other mustangs who are domesticated. I had a feral dog that learned everything from my other dog.
11. Self-soothe—whether it is chewing or licking, find a proactive way to turn an "anxiety" release into a simple self-soothe activity.
12. Time-out—everyone needs space. Honoring our animals in this way can be very healthy. Wolves and coyotes have a den, lions sleep in a pile—a lot, horses take turns napping while out in the wild. Everyone has a time-out where there is no pressure from each other. Unfortunately, we micromanage their lives, not realizing that they need to go nap in the other room. Going away for a while is good for them.

FOURTH CHAKRA EMOTIONS, SENSATIONS, AND QUESTIONS

Those emotions and sensations of the fourth chakra tend to rule their survival. Does your animal get to feel and express the full spectrum?

Fourth chakra emotions and sensations are:

- Heartfelt compassion
- Compassion for self
- Self-acceptance
- Unconditional love
- Neutral
- Wisdom
- Joy
- Grief
- Rage
- Panic
- Fear
- Bravery
- Hope
- Pride
- Anticipation
- Expectation
- Disappointment
- Defeat
- Content
- Willingness
- Devotion
- Loyalty
- Curiosity
- Childlike wonder

Ask yourself: Is your animal your soulmate or your heartmate?

FIFTH CHAKRA QUESTIONS

1. What is my animal's essence (persona, archetypes)?
2. What are my animal's favorite things (people, animals, activities, foods)?
3. Do they get to express this?
4. If so, how?
5. If not, how can I support more expression?

SIXTH CHAKRA QUESTIONS

1. Does my animal get to engage all their senses when they get out?
2. Does my animal "see" things?

SEVENTH CHAKRA QUESTIONS

1. Faith has a feeling. I have faith the sun will come up. I don't question that. Animals don't either. Does your animal feel like they have faith in you?
2. Does your animal feel like they have faith in others?
3. Is there something you can do to foster more of that?

EIGHTH CHAKRA QUESTIONS

1. Does your animal feel safe in their home environment?
2. Does your animal feel safe out in the world?
3. Does your animal feel connected to other animals?

CHAKRA DOMINANCE QUESTIONS

1. After reading all of what you wrote about your animal, is there a dominant chakra that could use some balancing?
2. Does your animal have one or two dominant chakras?
3. If so, what are they? (And do you see a correlation between the two dominant chakras?)

10

HEALING THE CHAKRAS

"Animal emotions are a matter of importance in their own right, but the very presence of animals—with their free-flowing emotions and empathy—is also critical to human well-being. Animal emotions should be important to us because we need animals in our lives; they help us. It's because animals have emotions that we're so drawn to them; lacking a shared language, emotions are perhaps our most effective means of cross-species communication. We can share our emotions, we can understand the language of feelings, and that's why we form deep and enduring social bonds with many other beings. Emotions are the glue that binds. They catalyze and regulate social interactions in animals and in humans."

—MARC BEKOFF, *From the Emotional Lives of Animals: A Leading Scientist Explores Animal Joy, Sorrow, and Empathy and Why They Matter*

Sharing Emotions, Sharing Lives is the chapter that I quoted above. And that is exactly what our household is, a vessel of shared lives and emotions.

In this chapter we dive into the world of animals in a different way. Feeling, sensing, and perceiving chakras has a whole different outcome than intellectual understanding. We gain insight into the chakra as a whole and see if there is a challenge to the whole being, or in one particular chakra—and see whether it is physical, emotional, or energetic. In the beginning, it is great to use tools like a pendulum. From there, if you keep practicing, you will have a sense of your animal in no time.

If you don't trust your intuition, you will have other tools until you get good at it and hopefully, that will lead to trusting yourself.

Techniques for Healing the Chakras

EXERCISE • GETTING STARTED

This is a simple technique to balance out the chakra system. When you think about what a perfect chakra would look like, picture this: it would be round, even, and spinning or vibrating at a consistent rate. Being aware of the shape and color of each chakra is important!

Also, I want you to imagine an hourglass.

A chakra is not a simple point but pervades the energetic and physical layers of the body, It opens towards two sides, the shape looking similar to an hourglass. The top part of the chakra would hover a little above the skin. The center of the hourglass would literally penetrate the organs that pertain to that particular chakra.

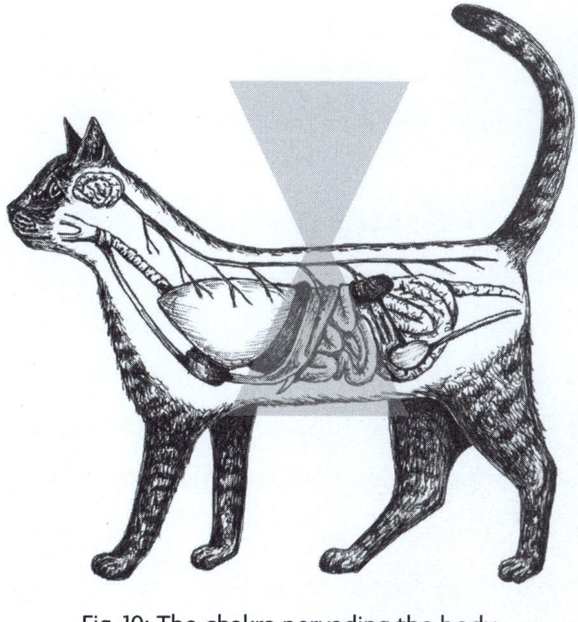

Fig. 10: The chakra pervading the body

Here is a rundown of the colors of each chakra:

- Root or 1st chakra—Red
- Sacral or 2nd chakra—Orange
- Solar Plexus or 3rd chakra—Yellow
- Heart or 4th chakra—Green
- Throat or 5th chakra—Blue
- Third Eye or 6th chakra—Purple, Indigo, or Violet
- Crown or 7th chakra—White

I want you to learn to spin the chakras in your mind's eye. But, before I teach you how, it's great to get a baseline of how each chakra is doing. I am going to use an exercise from my book *Energy Healing for Animals* to help with this:

You can experiment with a pendulum to see how your animal friend's chakras are doing. Hold the pendulum over a chakra and take note of whether the pendulum goes in a circular motion or back and forth, and if it's going in a circle, in what direction it is spinning (clockwise or counterclockwise). If you write down what you find, you can note the shift you have created after doing the chakra balancing technique.

EXERCISE • The Pendulum

The pendulum is an easy way to get a quick yes/no information and measure your work. It is a form of psychometry, a way of gaining information and measuring from the psyche. Galileo Galilei used the pendulum in the 1600s to keep time. Natural healer Hannah Kroeger wrote that since everything is a vibration, a pendulum is able to pick up on these vibrations.

A pendulum doesn't have to be fancy; in fact you can use a necklace, or you can go online and find something more elaborate with a crystal on the end. Basically, you could put anything on the end of a string or cord that weighs enough to swing and pivot – and you have your very own DIY pendulum.

- To get started, take the pendulum in one hand, and hold it over the other hand to get to know your pendulum and vibration. See how it responds to your empty palm. Is it moving back and forth? In circles?
- Next, you start to connect with your pendulum so you can create your "yes/no." You start by asking simple questions like, "Is my name Joan?" I will get a yes. You will get a no, unless your name is Joan also.
- From there, ask simple neutral questions such as: "Do I like asparagus?" "Is my front door red?" "Do I have a black dog?"

Keep playing with the yes and no questions until you feel confident that you trust what a yes is and what a no is. For you. Everyone is different. For me, yes swings forward and backward straight in front of me. A no swings from side to side. Some people get the exact opposite. Some people get a circle in one direction for a yes and a circle in the other direction for a no.

Before and After Picture

Before you start any healing work, the pendulum may indicate for you where you want to focus on for the animal's well-being, mentally, physically, and emotionally.

You can take the pendulum over each of the chakras (or an injured area) and see how the pendulum swings. Usually clockwise means optimum well-being.

Take notes based on your pendulum experience. Is it stopping over the chakra? Is it going backward? Is it going back and forth? Always stay neutral and write the information like data.

Once you perform the healing work and reset the chakras, you will be amazed at the difference of how the pendulum swings over the chakras!

Chakras on Cats and Puppies

In the Chakra Healing Kit link we have a video of checking the chakra on a cat. I was shocked that my cat Queen Latifah was so compliant. You may want to check the chakras on the chart (see color plates) as you will see in the video that cats and puppies may see this swinging thing as a toy and then all bets are off that you will get a clear read!

Here is the video on YouTube: ***https://www.youtube.com/watch?v=_Jp7S6VQvM8***

Even though you may think you know all that is going on with your animal companion, take a step back and objectively look at what the pendulum is telling you.

• • • • • • • • • • • • EXERCISE • Chakra Assessment • • • • • • • • • • • •

Print this worksheet out from my Chakra Healing Kit anytime you want to work on a new animal and assess their chakra health. You can use this before you do the balancing and then after you do the chakra balancing, or any other type of energy healing technique.

Whether I am doing animal communication or some form of energy healing, I do not "diagnose," I describe. I identify the size, shape, and speed along with the color vibrancy of the chakra.

You can find my Chakra Healing Kit here: ***https://joanranquet*** .com/product/animal-chakras-intro/

First Chakra

Before ______________________________

After ______________________________

Second Chakra

Before ______________________________

After ______________________________

Third Chakra

Before ______________________________

After ______________________________

Fourth Chakra

Before ______________________________

After ______________________________

Fifth Chakra

Before ______________________________

After ______________________________

Sixth Chakra

Before ______________________________

After ______________________________

Seventh Chakra

Before ______________________________

After ______________________________

Overall Field of Energy

Before ______________________________

After ______________________________

••••••••••• EXERCISE • Balancing the Chakras •••••••••••

You can do this on yourself first before you try it on another.

In the Chakra Healing Kit we have a recording. If you want to follow along with the recording: ***https://author.joanranquet.com/animal-chakra-healing/resources***

Get settled into a chair and feel into your whole body. Now, get a sense of your chakra system.

- Take a deep breath and feel your first chakra. Is it going clockwise? If not, try to get it to. Take note of the size, the shape, the speed at which it is moving, the color, and any other sense that you have about it.
- Take a deep breath and feel your second chakra. Is it going clockwise? If not, try to get it to. Take note of the size, the shape, the speed at which it is moving, the color, and any other sense that you have about it.
- Take a deep breath and feel your third chakra. Is it going clockwise? If not, try to get it to. Take note of the size, the shape, the speed at which it is moving, the color, and any other sense that you have about it.
- Take a deep breath and feel your fourth chakra. Is it going clockwise? If not, try to get it to. Take note of the size, the shape, the speed at which it is moving, the color, and any other sense that you have about it.
- Take a deep breath and feel your fifth chakra. Is it going clockwise? If not, try to get it to. Take note of the size, the shape, the speed at which it is moving, the color, and any other sense that you have about it.

- Take a deep breath and feel your sixth chakra. Is it going clockwise? If not, try to get it to. Take note of the size, the shape, the speed at which it is moving, the color, and any other sense that you have about it.
- Take a deep breath and feel your seventh chakra. Is it going clockwise? If not, try to get it to. Take note of the size, the shape, the speed at which it is moving, the color, and any other sense that you have about it.

Now, how do you feel?

Did you hear any tummy grumbling or experience any temperature change at any particular chakra? Raising your frequency and balancing out your chakras is a great place to start before working on others.

EXERCISE • Clockwise!

Now, get ready to balance the chakras of your animal companion.

Again, get comfortable. You can be touching the animal, or not. Always spin clockwise.

- In your mind's eye, I want you to see the first chakra of your animal companion. I want you to spin it. Get a sense of the size, the shape, the speed at which it is moving, the color, and any other thing you can determine. Work toward consistency.
- In your mind's eye, I want you to see the second chakra of your animal companion. I want you to spin it. Get a sense of the size, the shape, the speed at which it is moving, the color, and any other thing you can determine. Work toward consistency.

- In your mind's eye, I want you to see the third chakra of your animal companion. I want you to spin it. Get a sense of the size, the shape, the speed at which it is moving, the color, and any other thing you can determine. Work toward consistency.
- In your mind's eye, I want you to see the fourth chakra of your animal companion. I want you to spin it. Get a sense of the size, the shape, the speed at which it is moving, the color, and any other thing you can determine. Work toward consistency.
- In your mind's eye, I want you to see the fifth chakra of your animal companion. I want you to spin it. Get a sense of the size, the shape, the speed at which it is moving, the color, and any other thing you can determine. Work toward consistency.
- In your mind's eye, I want you to see the sixth chakra of your animal companion. I want you to spin it. Get a sense of the size, the shape, the speed at which it is moving, the color, and any other thing you can determine. Work toward consistency.
- In your mind's eye, I want you to see the seventh chakra of your animal companion. I want you to spin it. Get a sense of the size, the shape, the speed at which it is moving, the color, and any other thing you can determine. Work toward consistency.

You can get a sense of their overall well-being and their energy field. Now you can take a pendulum and go over the chakras again and see if it made any difference.

EXERCISE • Working Remotely

If the animal isn't right in front of you, you can still balance their chakras. You might print out the chart from the color plates and work as I do in this video: ***https://www.youtube.com/watch?v=_5bK16_48nI***

Once you have made your "before notes," then you can start the process again—it is the same:

- In your mind's eye, I want you to see the first chakra of your animal companion. I want you to spin it. Get a sense of the size, the shape, the speed at which it is moving, the color, and any other thing you can determine. Work toward consistency.
- In your mind's eye, I want you to see the second chakra of your animal companion. I want you to spin it. Get a sense of the size, the shape, the speed at which it is moving, the color, and any other thing you can determine. Work toward consistency.
- In your mind's eye, I want you to see the third chakra of your animal companion. I want you to spin it. Get a sense of the size, the shape, the speed at which it is moving, the color, and any other thing you can determine. Work toward consistency.
- In your mind's eye, I want you to see the fourth chakra of your animal companion. I want you to spin it. Get a sense of the size, the shape, the speed at which it is moving, the color, and any other thing you can determine. Work toward consistency.
- In your mind's eye, I want you to see the fifth chakra of your animal companion. I want you to spin it. Get a sense of the size, the shape, the speed at which it is moving, the

color, and any other thing you can determine. Work toward consistency.

- In your mind's eye, I want you to see the sixth chakra of your animal companion. I want you to spin it. Get a sense of the size, the shape, the speed at which it is moving, the color, and any other thing you can determine. Work toward consistency.
- In your mind's eye, I want you to see the seventh chakra of your animal companion. I want you to spin it. Get a sense of the size, the shape, the speed at which it is moving, the color, and any other thing you can determine. Work toward consistency.

You can get a sense of their overall well-being and their energy field. Now you can take a pendulum and go over the chakras again on the chart to see if it made any difference.

Finally . . .

You will get to a point where you won't necessarily need the pendulum. You'll just have a sense of the chakra's health on your own. In my Communication With All Life University (CWALU) classes, Energy Healing for Animals Fundamentals and Level 1, and my big program, Animal Mastery, eventually, medical intuition is developed enough to not use pendulums. It would be the same if you practiced this over and over again.

When I first started doing energy healing, I always made notes. It is a very good thing to watch over time. I always tell my students, when you have a journal of notes in which you check your progress, and you've been able to make a positive impact, that little journal becomes the "proof" of what you are doing. Having that physical proof is great for those days that you doubt your abilities, or if you don't have as much success with an animal.

Really take your time looking at all angles of the chakra. Don't get dead set on attaching an emotional value to a chakra that isn't quite working right. Or vice versa, don't get dead set on attaching a medical condition to a chakra.

For example, I regularly see students who quickly say that the throat chakra is small and not going very fast and therefore the animal must not be expressing themselves creatively. I always say, "Are you sure it isn't a thyroid issue? An allergy?" It is important to really be open and have a wide-eyed, childlike approach to see what shows up, rather than come to a conclusion right away.

I am really grateful that you are doing this work. This is rewarding for you and your animal companions. The more we have beings on the planet that are happy, healthy, and in a higher frequency, the more chance we have for harmony, peace, and well-being for all. Good vibes rub off!

For more information on live and self-paced courses and classes, visit: ***https://joanranquet.com/cwalu-courses/***

11 SUPPORT

"Domestication is something of a challenge to the cat; although ancient peoples took cats into their homes and hearts, their social life with humans has been very much love/hate since then, and it is much more recent in the cat's history than any other domestic animal that we finally 'brought in' for good. Our 'little cats' have a core of 'big cat' within them (as I'd noticed with the idea of tree and bush dwellers) and so they have similar needs in terms of behavior and health."

—JACKSON GALAXY, *Cat Daddy: What the World's Most Incorrigible Cat Taught Me About Life, Love and Coming Clean*

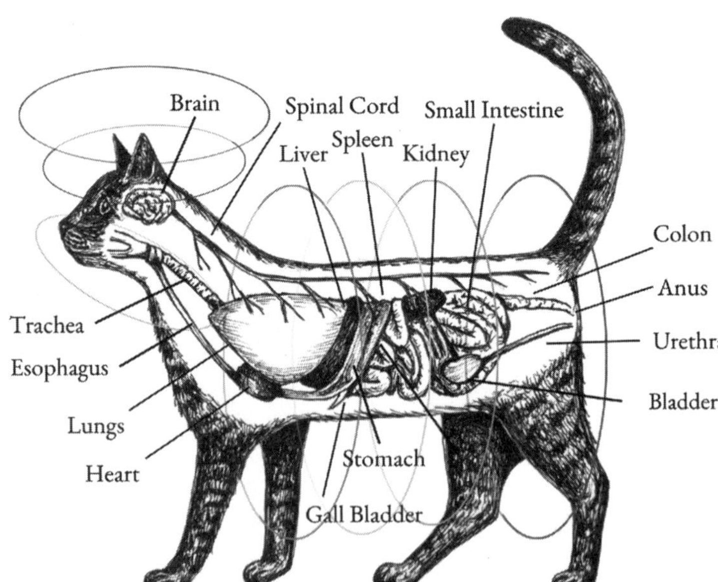

Fig. 11: Correlation of chakras and organs (see also the color plate)

Knowing more about the individual animal chakras and the areas they cover allows us to support our animals better. You find here some ideas on how to help with behavioural, emotional, and health challenges coming up in relation to each chakra.

First Chakra

Safety, supported, grounded, tribes, packs, herds, flocks, prides, colonies, immune system, safety, well-being, exercise.

How to help the first chakra with a behavioral or emotional issue

- Training
- Animal Communication
- Essential oils
- Bodywork or energy work
- Exercise

How to help the first chakra with a health challenge

- Immune building supplementation (feeding the immune/lymphatic system)
- Massage
- TTouch
- Flower essences
- Energy work

First chakra questions to ask yourself about your animal companion

1. Does your animal's fear show up in the physical stature?
2. If your animal has an immune system compromise, can you track back to an emotional experience that may have started this demise?

Second Chakra

One-on-one relationships, reproductive organs, creativity, play, joy, playfulness, abundance, desire, great relationships, and boundaries.

How to help the second chakra with a behavioral or emotional issue

- Animal communication
- Training
- Exercise
- Flower essences
- TTouch
- Fun

How to help the second chakra with a health challenge

- Cranio-sacral adjustment
- Acupuncture
- Acupressure
- Herbs
- Crystals
- Machines—healing devices, such as Rife Frequency Machines, PEMF (Pulsed Electromagnetic Field) Therapy, TheraPlate, etc.
- Healing Touch for Animals
- Energy work
- Feeding the elimination center/reproductive center

Second chakra questions to ask yourself about your animal companion

1. Does your animal companion have healthy, fun relationships with other animals?
2. As your animal companion has aged, does he/she still have creative outlets?

Third Chakra

Personal power, confidence, self-esteem, digestive organs, good food and supplementation.

How to help the third chakra with a behavioral or emotional issue

- Animal Communication
- Training
- Better diet
- Supplementation
- Flower essences

How to help the third chakra with a health challenge

- Chiropractic
- Pro/prebiotics
- Adjusting the diet/digestion
- Supplementation
- Homeopathy
- Feeding the digestive system/endocrine system

Third chakra questions to ask yourself about your animal companion

1. Do you notice when the animal's emotional anxiety is up, the digestion is off?
2. How can you find ways to help your animal companion experience more confidence in their own life? With you? With other humans? With other animals?

Fourth Chakra

Love, joy, grief, connection, forgiveness, understanding, heart and lungs, and great emotional environment.

How to help the fourth chakra with a behavioral or emotional issue

- Emotional environment—finding more joy
- Human emotional adjustments
- Flower essences
- Fun
- Exercise for all
- Animal Communication
- Training

How to help the fourth chakra with a health challenge

- Acupuncture
- Flower essences
- Massage
- Essential oils
- Feeding the cardiovascular/respiratory system

Fourth chakra questions to ask yourself about your animal companion

1. If your animal companion has experienced, or is experiencing, grief? Do you have some physical outlets for him/her to express and run some of it off?
2. If your animal companion is new to your household, do you have ways of helping him/her feel more comfortable and release old emotions from his prior household?

Fifth Chakra

Communicate, express, self-expression, the throat, and great purpose/job/integration.

How to help the fifth chakra with a behavioral or emotional issue

- Animal Communication
- Reframing picture for animal
- Find a new purpose
- Job
- Try new disciplines

How to help the fifth chakra with a health challenge

- Cranio-sacral adjustment
- Essential oils
- Adjusting the diet/digestion
- Herbs
- Digestive enzymes
- Feeding the will
- Redefining purpose

Fifth chakra questions to ask yourself about your animal companion

1. If your animal companion has a thyroid issue, was there ever a time that his/her emotional life was compromised?
2. Does your animal companion have a job/purpose in your household?

Sixth Chakra

Third eye, intuition, wisdom, intellect, pineal gland, senses, brain, and socialization with others of their species.

How to help the sixth chakra with a behavioral or emotional issue

- Training
- Outings

How to help the sixth chakra with a health challenge

- Cranial sacral
- Essential oils
- Homeopathy
- TTouch
- Feeding the senses, the brain, and the nervous system

Sixth chakra questions to ask yourself about your animal companion

1. Does your animal companion have healthy brain stimulation?
2. Does your animal companion have good outside stimulus?

Seventh Chakra

Divine connection crown, consciousness, trust, trust in humans, solid emotional leadership from one or more of their humans.

How to help the seventh chakra with a behavioral or emotional issue

- Dog training/horse training for humans
- Human works on improving their own self-esteem

How to help the seventh chakra with a health challenge

- Cranio-sacral adjustment
- TTouch
- Supplementation/feeding the skeletal/musculature system, and getting a flow through all the meridians

Seventh chakra questions to ask yourself about your animal companion

1. Does your animal companion trust humans?
2. Do you trust your animal companion?

Eighth Chakra

Grace, the aura of the collective ecosystem for that animal, specific species and/or the home of the morphic resonance, ecosystems, the energy of the whole has a signature feel of harmony.

How to help the eighth chakra with a behavioral or emotional issue

1. Feng shui
2. Healing Touch
3. Scalar wave energy
4. Space clearing

How to help the eighth chakra with a health challenge

1. Energy work
2. Creating a state of grace
3. Feeding and supporting the emotional system of the whole body, and the environment

Eighth chakra questions to ask yourself about your animal companion

- Does your household feel safe?
- Do you need to put energetic bubbles up so your animal companions don't take on too much of your "stuff"?
- How many animals feel familiar? Are they being "called into" this ecosystem, maybe not just for you but for others in the family?

A FINAL WORD

All the classes, products, and services in the world can only go so deep. There is no better way to understand your animal than diving into their emotional, physical, mental, energetic, species-specific, and spiritual blueprint. Whether it is animal communication, energy healing, or energetic support, practice makes perfect.

Continually asking yourself all the questions in the last three chapters will help you to unravel the biggest mysteries.

As we've examined throughout this entire book, seeing things from an animal's perspective is what will truly make a difference to their lives. We can think of it from our own perspective all day long. But when we look at them in this different light, we start to shift things for them.

Ultimately our emotional leadership is what keeps our animals in our home happy and thriving. Having good habits for grounding become very helpful when we are challenged in all directions.

I'm very excited for you to take this big leap.

RESOURCES

Wheels of Light: Chakras, Auras, and the Healing Energy of the Body, Rosalyn L. Bruyere (A Fireside Book, 1989)

Wheels of Life: A User's Guide to the Chakra System, Anodea Judith, Ph.D. (Llewellyn Publications, 1987)

Unblocked, A Revolutionary Approach to Tapping into Your Chakra Empowerment Energy to Reclaim Your Passion, Joy, and Confidence, Margaret Lynch Raniere and David Raniere, Ph.D. (Hay House, 2021)

Chakra Awakening: Transform Your Reality Using Crystals, Color, Aromatherapy & the Power of Positive Thought, Margaret Ann Lembo (Llewellyn Publications, 2011)

Anatomy of the Spirit: The Seven Stages of Power and Healing, Caroline Myss, Ph.D. (Bantam, 1997)

Hands of Light: A Guide to Healing Through the Human Energy Field, Barbara Ann Brennan (Bantam, 1988)

The Wonder of Unicorns: Ascending with the Higher Angelic Realms, Diana Cooper (Findhorn Press, 2019)

An Immense World: How Animal Senses Reveal the Hidden Realms Around Us, Ed Yong (Random House, 2022)

Horse Brain, Human Brain: The Neuroscience of Horsemanship, Janet L. Jones, Ph.D. (Trafalgar Square, 2020)

Through a Dog's Ear: Using Sound to Improve the Health and Behavior of Your Canine Companion, Joshua Leeds, Susan Wagner (Sounds True, 2008)

The Elephant's Secret Sense: The Hidden Life of the Wild Herds of Africa, Caitlin O'Connell (University of Chicago Press; Reprint edition, 2008)

Living Buddha, Living Christ, Thich Nhat Hanh (Riverhead Books, 1995)

Cat Daddy: What the World's Most Incorrigible Cat Taught Me About Life, Love and Coming Clean, Jackson Galaxy, (Penguin Publishing Group, 2013)

Animal Speak: The Spiritual & Magical Powers of Creatures Great & Small, Ted Andrews (Llewellyn Publications, 1993)

INDEX

ABOUT THE AUTHOR

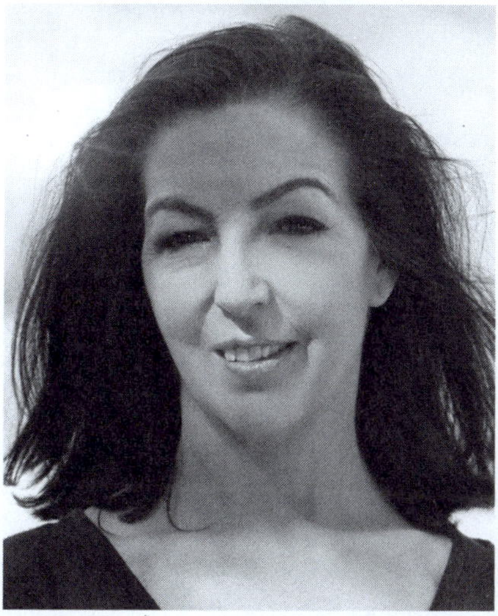

Photo by Dan Frenkel

Joan Ranquet is an inspired animal communicator, energy healer, and educator. The founder of the Communication With All Life University (CWALU), an experiential learning platform for animal communication, energy healing, nature and wildlife, she teaches through workshops, wildlife retreats, and private sessions.

Passionate about animals all her life, Joan is the author of several books, including *Emotional Freedom Technique for Animals and Their Humans*, *Energy Healing for Animals*, and *Communication with All Life*. Her TEDx talk, "The Rainbow Bridge: Animals in Transition," received more than 474,000 views on YouTube.

Joan lives in Santa Clarita, California, with her animal family of four horses, three dogs, and three cats.

For further information visit: ***https://joanranquet.com***.

